Gonioscopy

Christoph Faschinger • Anton Hommer

Gonioscopy

Springer

Authors
Prof. Christoph Faschinger
Medical University Graz
Graz
Austria

Dr. Anton Hommer
"Sanatorium Hera"
Glaucoma Outpatient Service Hospital
Vienna
Austria

ISBN 978-3-642-28609-4 ISBN 978-3-642-28610-0 (eBook)
DOI 10.1007/978-3-642-28610-0
Springer Heidelberg New York Dordrecht London

Library of Congress Control Number: 2012938652

Printed on acid-free paper

Springer is part of Springer Science+Business Media (www.springer.com)

I dedicate this book to Günter K. Krieglstein, Professor emeritus, Cologne, Germany, with many thanks. He was always a wonderful teacher and an outstanding and helpful personality during my ophthalmological career. Let's call him a "prime number person".

Christoph Faschinger

This book is dedicated to my father, Kurt Hommer, Professor for Ophthalmology in Vienna and Linz. Thus I had the opportunity in my childhood to meet some of the famous ophthalmologists from the past in our home: H. Goldmann, A. Franceschetti, J. Francois, W. Leydhecker, J. Fronimopoulos and F. Fankhauser are just a few. Perhaps, besides the "genetic risk factor", this was the reason why I chose ophthalmology and especially glaucoma as my "subspecialty".
My father's long experience and personal teaching in ophthalmology and glaucoma was always of great help to me and had a significant influence on my ophthalmological work.

Anton Hommer

Foreword

The human eye offers the unique advantage that most of its structures can be visualized and inspected for diagnostic purposes in health and disease. Gonioscopy – an indispensable key element in the work-up of glaucoma – benefits considerably from this fact, which is elegantly reviewed in the present book. Its comprehensive and well-structured chapters together with superb illustrations make it a textbook and an atlas at the same time.

All aspects of gonioscopy are covered, starting with the history of gonioscopy and examination techniques, followed by anatomical and developmental features as well as grading systems. Typical gonioscopic findings in open-angle glaucoma and angle-closure glaucomas – presented as high-quality goniophotographs – mirror the clinical experience of the two authors. The chapter on imaging techniques supplementary to gonioscopy is particularly interesting. The effect of therapy (laser, surgery, medication) on the appearance of the chamber angle is another highlight of this publication. The index at the end of the book is adequately detailed and enables quick finding and orientation on special issues.

This book on gonioscopy is certainly a helpful and most competent companion for everyone who is entrusted with the care of glaucoma patients. It has brought together an impressive selection of photographically well-documented findings in the chamber angle of many clinical forms of glaucoma. A reasonable number of tables contributes to the systematic overview of this special field of ophthalmology.

It must have been a demanding task for the authors to put together this fine book with all its relevant illustrations; however, the outcome is a fitting reflection of their commitment and effort. We congratulate both authors of this book which is immensely useful for both the community of ophthalmologists and the glaucoma patients they are taking care of.

I sincerely wish that this publication becomes widely consulted for the above reasons as a significant tool for achieving success in the differential diagnosis of glaucomas.

Cologne, Germany G.K. Krieglstein

Preface

Do you remember your ophthalmology teacher? Sitting at the slit lamp, a lens in his/her hand, rotating slowly clockwise, staring into the tubes of the slit lamp and the patient waiting patiently for the end of the procedure while methylcellulose ran down his/her cheek … and no words, a few notes, maybe a small sketch. And you have been standing watching, seeking information, desiring to do the gonioscopy yourself to get an insight into these delicate parts of the eye. No chance, next time, maybe, …

Gonioscopy was not always taught in former times. But new classifications (of angle closure) and new methods of surgery directly targeting the cause of primary open angle glaucoma, the pathological trabecular meshwork, aroused increasing interest. Educational courses are offered at meetings, the internet provides more and more information and: this new book has been prepared to recall and complete your knowledge about the chamber angle and gonioscopy.

The aim of gonioscopy is to distinguish between normal aspects and their variations and between changes due to aging or caused by different pathologies. The initial therapy is totally different in an open and a closed angle!

Gonioscopy is a simple technique, easy to learn, but it needs experience. So do it as often as possible; it is very satisfying, it gives you a lot of information, it is a necessity for arriving at an appropriate diagnosis and for deciding on an adequate therapy. It is really worth doing it! Start today!

We wish you an entertaining reading and much success with your glaucoma patients!

Christoph Faschinger
Anton Hommer

Acknowledgements

Almost all figures and drawings are from the University Eye Clinic Graz. They were done by our photographers H. Bauer, R. Kim and S. Strohmayer, to whom we are extremely grateful.

Many thanks to Springer-Verlag, especially to Ms. I. Bohn for her friendly and professional administrative support, to Mr. I.S. Vignesh, project manager, for his perfect and outstanding layout work, and to Mr. S. Klemp, who was responsible for the realization of this book project.

Contents

1 History of Gonioscopy 1
Bibliography 3

2 How to Perform Gonioscopy 5
2.1 Lenses 5
2.2 Regular Procedure 5
2.3 Dynamic or Indentation Gonioscopy 8
2.4 Surroundings 9
2.5 Tonometry or Gonioscopy: Which First? 9
2.6 Importance of Gonioscopy 9
Bibliography 10

3 Anatomical Structures of the Chamber Angle 11
3.1 Schwalbe's Line or Ring 11
3.2 Trabecular Meshwork 12
3.3 Schlemm's Canal 14
3.4 Scleral Spur 15
3.5 Anterior Ciliary Muscle Band 15
3.6 Iris Root and Iris 16
3.7 Posterior Ciliary Muscle Band, Ciliary Sulcus 21
3.8 Blood Vessels 22
3.9 Sampaolesi's Line 22
3.10 Lens 22
3.11 Cornea 23
3.12 Decision Tree 23
Bibliography 23

4 Development of the Chamber Angle and Developmental Disorders 25
4.1 Embryology of the Parts of the Chamber Angle 25
4.2 Examples of Genetic Disorders of the Anterior Segment . . . 27
4.2.1 Primary Congenital Glaucoma, Hydrophthalmus, Buphthalmus, Childhood Glaucoma (Birth to the 10th Year of Life) 27
4.2.2 More Complex Dysgeneses: Secondary Childhood Glaucomas 28
Bibliography 29

5 **Grading Systems and Documentation** ... 31
5.1 Gonioscopic Grading Systems ... 31
5.1.1 Scheie ... 31
5.1.2 Shaffer ... 31
5.1.3 Shaffer ... 32
5.1.4 Spaeth ... 32
5.1.5 Becker ... 33
5.1.6 Shaffer-Kanski ... 33
5.2 Non-gonioscopic Grading Systems ... 34
5.2.1 Peripheral Anterior Chamber (Van Herick Method) ... 34
5.2.2 Central Anterior Chamber (Ghorbani-Smith Method) ... 34
5.2.3 Additional Procedures in Gonioscopy ... 36
5.3 Documentation of the Structures of the Chamber Angle ... 36
Bibliography ... 37

6 **Open Angle and Glaucoma** ... 39
6.1 The Chamber Angle in Primary Open-Angle Glaucoma or Ocular Hypertension with Open Angle ... 39
6.2 The Chamber Angle in Secondary Open-Angle Glaucoma ... 39
6.2.1 Open-Angle Glaucoma Caused by Ocular Diseases ... 39
6.2.2 Open-Angle Glaucoma Caused by Extraocular Diseases ... 46
6.2.3 Iatrogenic Open-Angle Glaucoma ... 47
Bibliography ... 48

7 **Angle Closure and Glaucoma** ... 49
7.1 The Chamber Angle in Primary Angle-Closure Disease ... 49
7.1.1 Risk Factors ... 49
7.1.2 Terminology and Classification of Morphological and Functional Changes ... 50
7.1.3 Terms ... 51
7.1.4 Classification of the Causes of Angle Closure ... 51
7.1.5 Acute Angle Closure (Attack) ... 55
7.1.6 Status Post-Acute Angle-Closure (Attack) ... 57
7.1.7 Management of Angle-Closure Disease ... 58
7.2 The Chamber Angle in Secondary Angle Closure ... 58
7.2.1 Causes of Secondary Angle Closure ... 59
Bibliography ... 62

8 **Additional Examinations to Gonioscopy** ... 65
8.1 AS-OCT ... 65
8.2 UBM ... 66
8.3 Pentacam-Scheimpflug ... 67
8.4 Orbscan ... 67
8.5 EyeCam ... 67
Bibliography ... 68

9 Laser Treatments in the Chamber Angle 69
9.1 Thermal Lasers 69
9.1.1 Laser trabeculoplasty. 69
9.1.2 Argon Laser Suturolysis 69
9.1.3 Argon Laser Peripheral Iridoplasty 69
9.1.4 Transscleral Cyclophotocoagulation 70
9.1.5 Endoscopic Cyclophotocoagulation, Endocycloplasty 71
9.2. Non-thermal Lasers 71
9.2.1 Selective Laser Trabeculoplasty 71
9.3 Disruptive Lasers. 72
9.4 Excimer Lasers 72
Bibliography 73

10 Surgery in the Chamber Angle 75
10.1 Filtration or Penetrating Surgery (Trabeculectomy) 75
10.2 Non-penetrating Surgery 75
10.2.1 Deep Sclerectomy 75
10.2.2 Viscocanalostomy 76
10.2.3 Viscotrabeculotomy. 76
10.3 Implants. 77
10.3.1 Canaloplasty 77
10.3.2 iStent Trabecular Micro-Bypass 77
10.3.3 Ex-PRESS Mini Glaucoma Shunt. 77
10.3.4 SOLX Gold Shunt
10.3.5 Tube Shunts. 77
10.4 Trabeculectomy Ab Interno. 78
10.5 Trabeculotomy, Goniotomy 78
10.6 Surgery of the Ciliary Body: Cyclodialysis 78
10.7 Peripheral Iridectomy 79
Bibliography 79

11 Influences of Medications on the Chamber Angle 81
11.1 Increase in IOP Induced by Steroids. 81
11.2 Angle Closure Induced by Drugs 81
11.2.1 Direct Sympathomimetic, Adrenergic Drugs 81
11.2.2 Indirect Sympathomimetic Drugs 81
11.2.3 Parasympatholytic, Anticholinergic Drugs 82
11.2.4 Selective Serotonin Reuptake Inhibitors 82
11.2.5 Other Drugs Without Pupillary Block. 82
Bibliography 82

Index. 83

Abbreviations

AAC	Acute angle-closure attack
ACD	Anterior chamber depth
ACV	Anterior chamber volume
ALPI	Argon Laser peripheral iridoplasty
ALT	Argon Laser trabeculoplasty
AOD	Angle opening distance
ARA	Angle recess area
AS-OCT	Anterior segment optical coherence tomography
COCO	Controlled coagulation
CYP1B1	Cytochrome P 450 1B1
DLT	Diode Laser trabeculoplasty
ECP	Endoscopic cyclophotocoagulation
ECPL	Endocycloplasty
ELT	Excimer Laser trabeculoplasty
GMS	Gold micro shunt
HLA-B27	Human leucocyte antigene B27
ICE syndrome	Irido-corneal-endothelial syndrome
ILC	Irido-lenticular contact area
IOP	Intraocular pressure
ITC	Irido-trabecular contact
LE	Left eye
LPI	Laser peripheral iridotomy
LTBP2	Latent transforming growth factor beta binding protein 2
LTP	Laser trabeculoplasty
μm	Micrometer
min	Minute
mJ	MilliJoule
mm	Millimeter
ms	Millisecond
mW	Milliwatt
Nd:YAG	Neodymium:Yttrium-Aluminium-Garnet
nm	Nanometer
ns	Nanosecond
OAG	Open-angle glaucoma
OTC	Over-the-counter
OVD	Ophthalmic viscous device
PAC	Primary angle closure
PACG	Primary angle-closure glaucoma
PACS	Primary angle-closure suspect

PAS	Peripheral anterior synechia(e)
PDS	Pigment dispersion syndrome
PG	Pigment dispersion glaucoma
POAG	Primary open-angle glaucoma
PXG	Pseudoexfoliation glaucoma
PXS	Pseudoexfoliation syndrome
RE	Right eye
RNFL	Retinal nerve fibre layer
s	Second
SLT	Selective Laser trabeculoplasty
SS	Scleral spur
TIA	Trabecular-iris angle
TIGR gene	Trabecular meshwork glucocorticoid response gene
TISA	Trabecular-iris spur area
TM	Trabecular meshwork
TSCPC	Transscleral cyclophotocoagulation
UBM	Ultrasound biomicroscopy
X-ray	Electromagnetic radiation

1 History of Gonioscopy

As a member of the board of Ophthalmology at the University Eye Clinic Graz since 1978. I – by chance – served at the same University where Maximilian Salzmann (Fig. 1.1; born 1862 in Vienna, Austria and died 1954 in Graz, Austria) was professor and chairman from 1911 to 1932. Salzmann was the first to use a contact lens (originally designed for correction of irregular astigmatism) and indirect gonioscopy for examination of the chamber angle besides direct observations. He produced wonderful detailed paintings of the chamber angle and the observed pathologies (Figs. 1.2 and 1.3).

Independently, and some years before, Alexios Trantas (born 1867 in Konitsa, Greece, and died 1961 in Istanbul, Turkey) coined the word "gonioscopy". *Gonia* means "angle" and *skopein* means to "observe" in Greek. He described the chamber angle using a direct ophthalmoscope and simultaneous digital pressure on the limbal region. Therefore both scientists are called "fathers of gonioscopy".

Further pioneers were M. U. Troncoso (anatomical structures), T. Thornburn (peripheral anterior synechiae, photography of the angle), O. Barkan (differentiation between open-angle glaucoma (OAG), narrow-angle glaucoma and the first description of goniotomy).

An important step forward was the invention of a practicable slit lamp with magnification, powerful illumination and stereoscopic view. In a study reported in 1956, Shaffer and Tour compared the formerly used gonioscopic methods, and drew the following conclusion: "the easiest and least confusing gonioscopic method for beginners, and perhaps for the average ophthalmologist, is the use of a 16-mm glass Koeppe contact lens, the Barkan hand illuminator, and the hand-held Haag-Streit gonioscopic microscope."

In particular, Goldmann's gonioscopes (a one mirror and later a three-mirror lens) made the

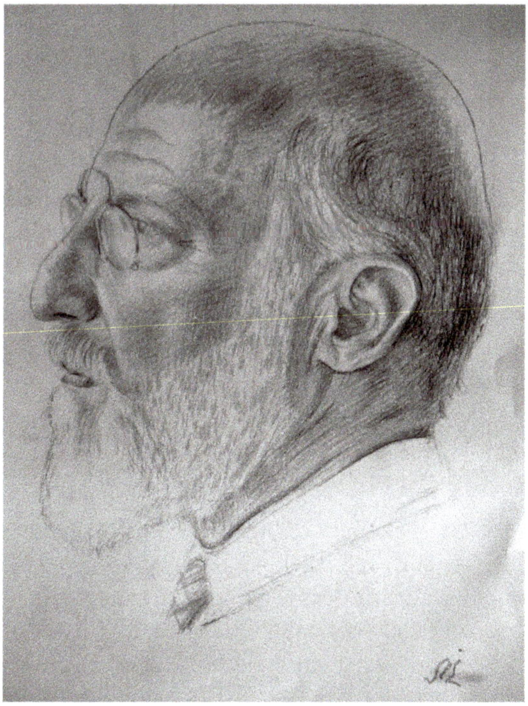

Fig. 1.1 Portrait of Maximilian Salzmann

C. Faschinger, A. Hommer, *Gonioscopy*,
DOI 10.1007/978-3-642-28610-0_1, © Springer-Verlag Berlin Heidelberg 2012

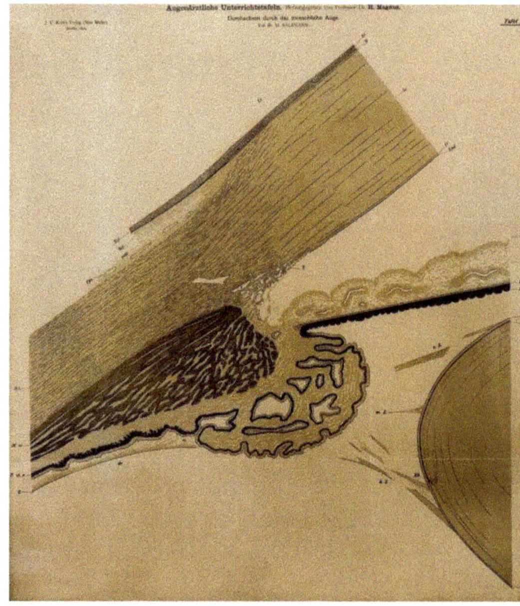

Fig. 1.2 Salzmann's painting of a normal chamber angle. Note the detail! The angle is open, the iris insertion is deep at the ciliary body, the iris configuration is flat, the angularity is 35°. The posterior ciliary sulcus and the ciliary body, the zonular fibers with the lens, the longitudinal and radial fibers of the ciliary muscle, sclera and cornea, Schlemm's canal, an intrascleral vessel and the trabecular meshwork are easily seen

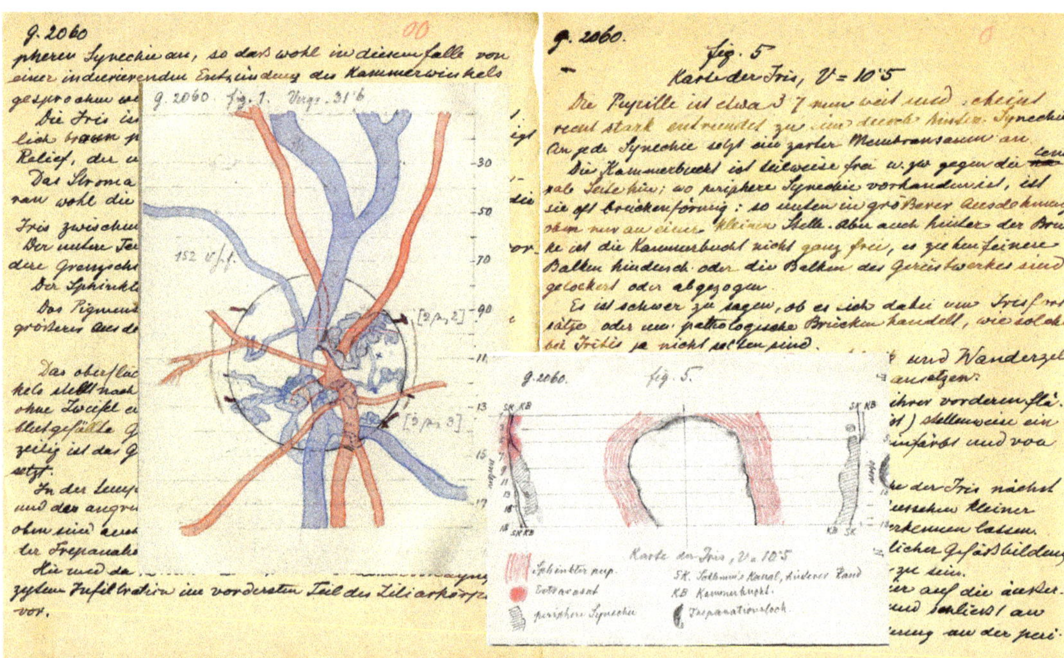

Fig. 1.3 Drawings of the disc (with collaterals), the iris (the sphincter pupillae is colored *red*) with the chamber angle (peripheral synechiae are in *gray*) and Salzmann's hand-written description of the histological findings in an eye with neovascular glaucoma after central venous thrombosis. Original text: "The chamber angle is not free, there are fine arbors crossing … it is difficult to say, if these are iris processes or pathological bridges …"

examination much easier. We still perform the examination in the same way as he described with the patient sitting at the slit lamp and a lens on the eye rotated 360° by the examiner.

Grading systems, especially that of Spaeth, and the introduction of dynamic gonioscopy (Forbes) made the classification of different glaucomas comprehensible and reproducible. Findings from sophisticated machines such as anterior segment optical coherence tomography (AS-OCT) and ultrasound biomicroscopy (UBM) offered important insights into specific mechanisms.

Detailed histories of gonioscopy by Dellaporta and Alward are available, and are worth reading.

Bibliography

Alward WLM (2011) A history of gonioscopy. Optom Vis Sci 88:29–35

Dellaporta A (1975) Historical notes on gonioscopy. Surv Ophthalmol 20:137–149

Forbes M (1966) Gonioscopy with corneal indentation. Arch Ophthalmol 76:488–492

Goldmann H (1938) Zur Technik der Spaltlampenmikroskopie. Ophthalmologica 96:90–97

Salzmann M (1914) Die Ophthalmoskopie der Kammerbucht. Z Augenheilk 31:1–19

Shaffer RN, Tour RL (1956) A comparative study of gonioscopic methods. Am J Ophthalmol 41:256–265

Spaeth GL (1971) The normal development of the human anterior chamber angle: a new system of descriptive grading. Trans Ophthalmol Soc U K 91:709–739

Sugar HS, Foster CC (1981) Maximilian Salzmann. Ophthalmic pioneer and artist. Surv Ophthalmol 26:28–30

How to Perform Gonioscopy

2

Gonioscopy is an examination usually performed in a sitting person at the slit lamp (Fig. 2.1). Only during glaucoma surgery or for examinations under general anesthesia in babies or in sedated infants does the patient lie in a supine position (Fig. 2.2).

2.1 Lenses

The structures of the chamber angle are only visible with lenses put on the eye, because light rays coming from the chamber angle are totally absorbed by inner reflections by the cornea. The lens on the cornea has a higher refractive index than the cornea and the tear fluid.

For surgery the surgeon may use a very thick, convex lens for *direct* gonioscopy (a Koeppe lens, or a Swan Jacob lens; Fig. 2.3).

Indirect gonioscopy as a routine examination is performed with lenses that have a different numbers of mirrors located at variable angles. The Goldmann three-mirror lens is the best known and most popular one. For gonioscopy the smallest mirror with the steepest angle is used. All these lenses have a diameter larger than that of the cornea (15 mm in adults). The curvature of the lenses is steeper than that of a regular cornea, so some contact gel (methylcellulose) is needed between the lens and the cornea.

Lenses for *dynamic* or *indentation* gonioscopy have a smaller diameter than that of the cornea (9 mm). Their curvature is (almost) the same as that of a regular cornea so no contact gel is needed for examination. They are indispensable for differential diagnoses in angle-closure pathologies (Figs. 2.4 and 2.5).

2.2 Regular Procedure

Always explain to the patient what you are going to do!
Always examine both eyes!

First anesthetize the eyes with a drop of topical anesthetic applied into the cul-de-sac of the lower conjunctiva. Use enough contact gel on the concave part of the lens, fill up that hollow and avoid air bubbles. Ask the patient to open both eyes and to look upwards, take a cotton-stick to pull the lower lid downwards (Fig. 2.6) and place the lens

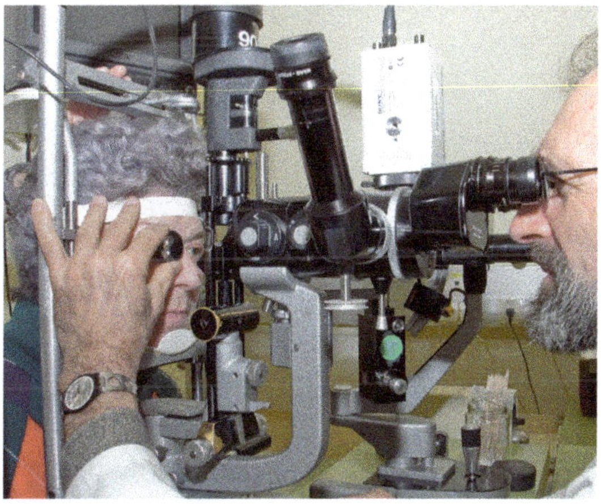

Fig. 2.1 Patient sitting at the slit lamp for gonioscopy (Goldmann three-mirror lens)

C. Faschinger, A. Hommer, *Gonioscopy*,
DOI 10.1007/978-3-642-28610-0_2, © Springer-Verlag Berlin Heidelberg 2012

gently with its lower edge into the lower cul-de-sac, then tilt the lens with the contact fluid onto the cornea (Fig. 2.7). Sometimes the upper lid interferes in patients who squeeze their lids and you have to repeat the procedure.

Ask the patient to look straight ahead. Remember, the part of the chamber angle that you examine is 180° away from the position of the mirror you use.

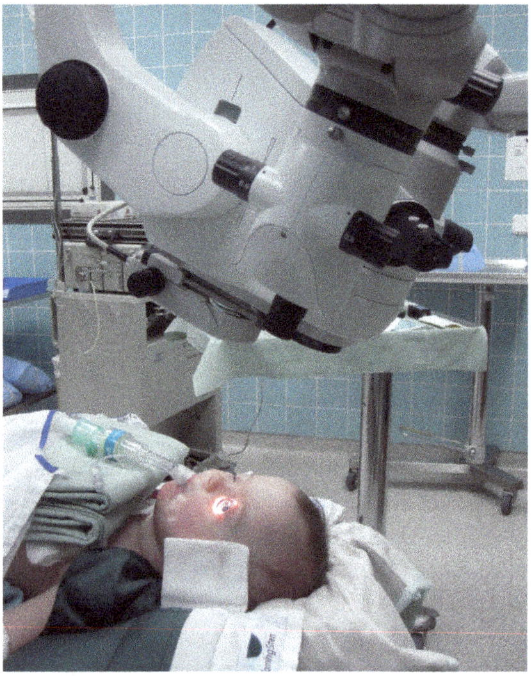

Fig. 2.2 Baby lying under a microscope in the operating room for gonioscopy (Koeppe lens). The microscope is tilted to 45° to get a good view of the structures of the angle

Start with the inferior angle (Fig. 2.8)!

The superior angle is always a bit narrower than the inferior angle, probably due to the pressure of the upper lid. The pigmentation of the inferior angle is usually more prominent due to hydrostatics. Therefore, it is easier to identify the structures in the inferior angle. Rotate the lens to bring the smallest mirror to the 12 o'clock position. Then adjust the slit lamp to 0° and examine the chamber angle clockwise (better than counter-clockwise, because you will remember the pathological changes according to the clock hours more easily). Start with low

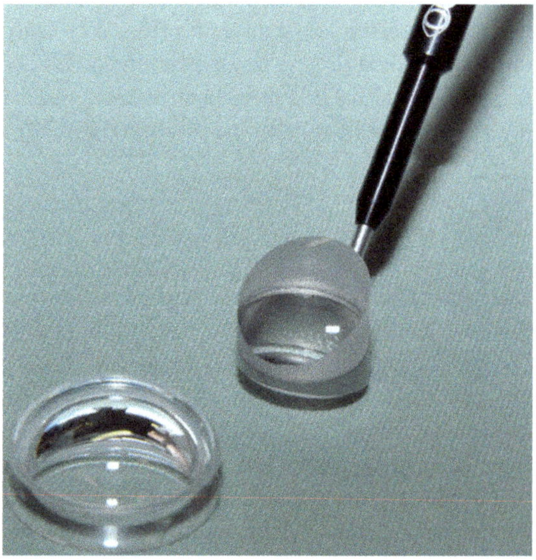

Fig. 2.3 Lenses for direct gonioscopy: Koeppe lens (*left*), Swan Jacob lens with handle (*right*)

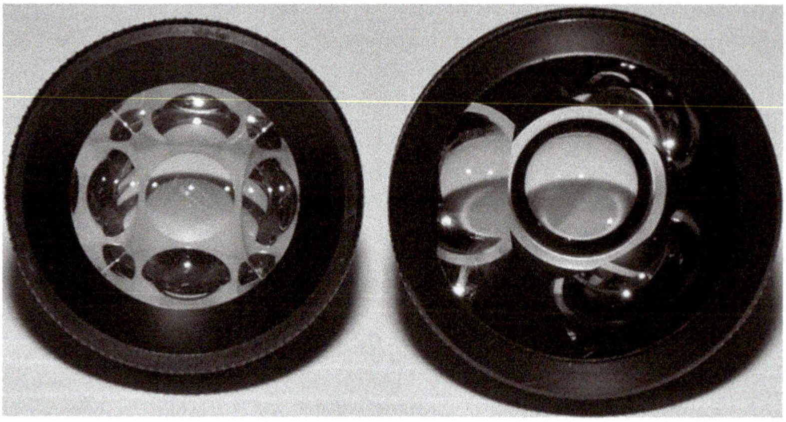

Fig. 2.4 Lenses for gonioscopy: Sussman four-mirror lens for dynamic gonioscopy (*left*), Goldmann three-mirror lens for regular gonioscopy

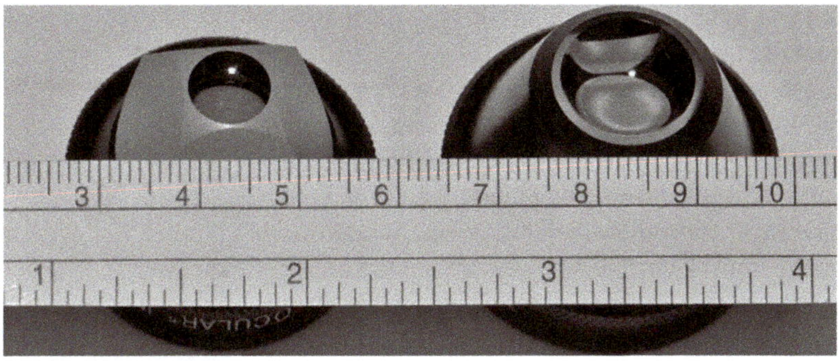

Fig. 2.5 Sussman lens with a diameter smaller than the cornea and a Goldmann lens with a diameter larger then the cornea (*upper scale* millimeters, *lower scale* inches)

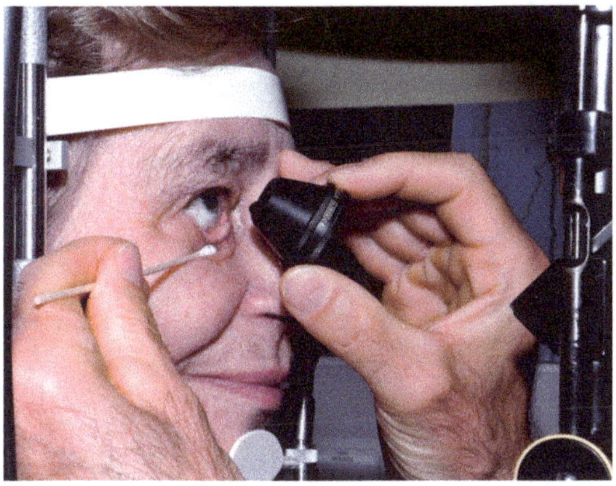

Fig. 2.6 The patient is asked to look upwards. A cotton stick is used to pull down the lower lid and the lens is placed gently with its lower edge in the lower cul-de-sac

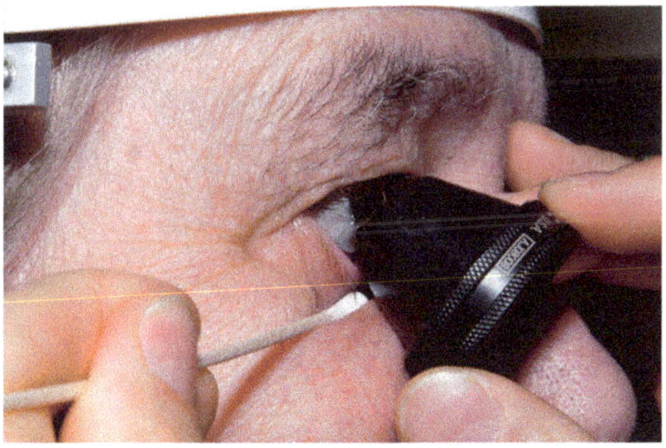

Fig. 2.7 The lens is tilted with the contact fluid onto the cornea

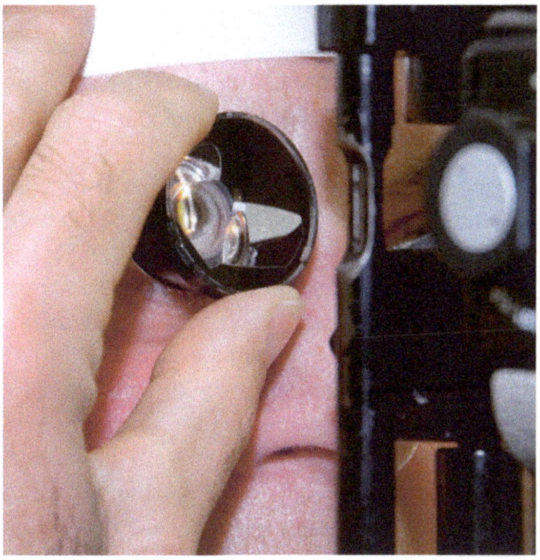

Fig. 2.8 The smallest mirror of the Goldmann three-mirror lens is at the 12 o'clock position, ready to examine the inferior angle

magnification and change to a higher one if you want to see more detail.

Be sure to keep in mind your findings and document them correctly. After you have finished your first 360° examination, perform a second examination with different magnifications and/or light conditions. Start with a bright beam to get an overview, use a narrow beam for the corneal "wedge" to identify Schwalbe's ring. Dim the light in a narrow angle, otherwise constriction of the pupil will pull out the iris from the angle so that the angle appears wider than it really is.

At the end of the examination ask the patient to squeeze the lids firmly. The lens will come off the cornea easily. Afterwards you should wash out the remnants of the contact gel of the eye with saline solution. The lens should be properly sterilized for the next patient.

Try to perform your first gonioscopies under the supervision of an experienced person via the second tube of the slit lamp or via videotaping, and discuss your findings.

In a narrow angle, you can ask the patient to look towards the direction of the steepest mirror. You keep the lens in the frontal position without a tilt. Now the beam will go over the iris and into the angle for a more detailed view. In addition, the margin of the lens will provide some pressure on the cornea or limbus and will push the aqueous humor into the opposite part of the angle. Therefore this part will become slightly wider than it really is. Keep this in mind!

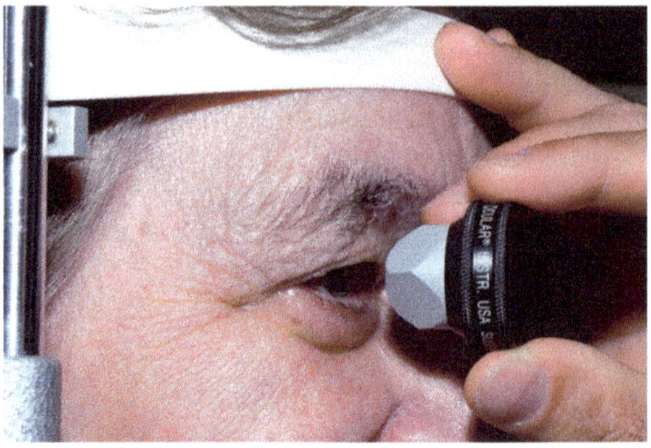

Fig. 2.9 Indentation or dynamic gonioscopy with a lens of contact diameter less than the cornea. Contact fluid such as methylcellulose is not necessary because the curvature of the lens and the cornea are the same

2.3 Dynamic or Indentation Gonioscopy

In eyes with a closed angle you have to distinguish between an iridotrabecular contact (ITC, apposition) and peripheral anterior synechiae (PAS). The proper therapy depends strongly on these findings.

For better differentiation, the use of a lens with a smaller diameter than the cornea (9 mm) is mandatory. There are lenses with and without a handle. Try both types and decide which you prefer. Anesthetize the eyes and wait for a short while. Because the lens has a smaller diameter and a curvature similar to that of the cornea, no contact fluid is needed. Ask the patient to look straight ahead and put the lens gently on the surface of the cornea. You do not have to rotate it, because all four mirrors have the same angularity. To get a 360° view you only have to change the position of the slit beam (Fig. 2.9).

Initially you may not find all of the structures of the chamber angle because the iris is bowed forward. You may be able to identify Schwalbe's ring and the anterior parts of the trabecular meshwork (Shaffer grade 2). Indentation of the globe by applying gentle pressure to the cornea will change the fluid compartment in the anterior chamber and will widen the angle. An ITC or apposition will open and you will be able to see more detail of the chamber angle. A synechia will remain unchanged and the chamber angle will stay the same in that particular part (Figs. 2.10 and 2.11).

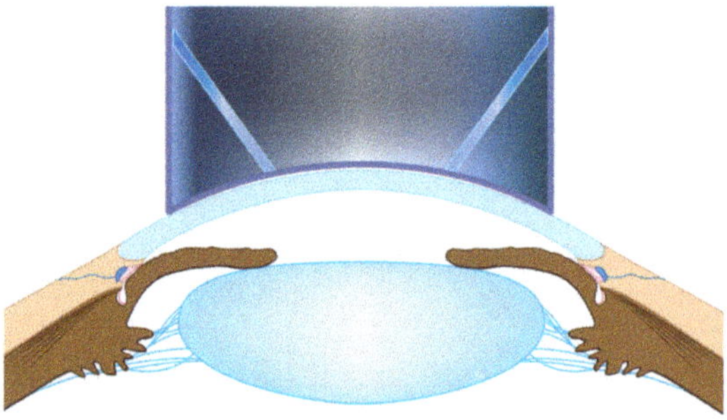

Fig. 2.10 Schematic drawing showing a closed angle due to contact of the iris to the trabecular meshwork before indentation gonioscopy with a lens of diameter smaller than the cornea

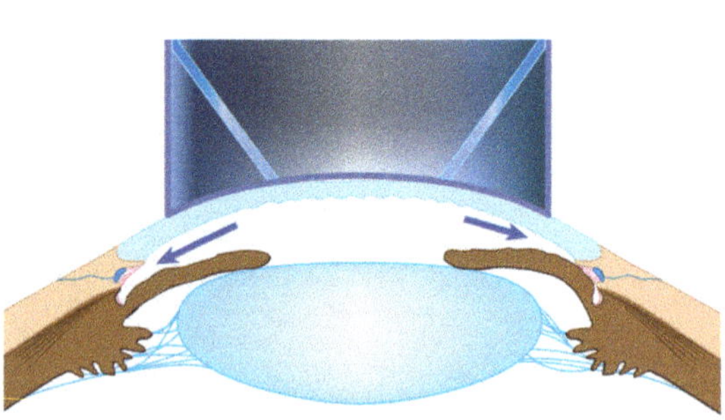

Fig. 2.11 Schematic drawing showing the chamber angle during indentation gonioscopy: the ITC has opened (*left angle*), the synechia remains unchanged and closes the angle (*right angle*)

Examine the chamber angle with all four mirrors and document your findings. It makes an important difference to the therapy if less or more than 270° is closed or not. If the applied pressure is too high, corneal folds will appear and will worsen your view. Therefore, practice applying pressure since an understanding of how much pressure to apply has to be gained by experience. Be very gentle and do not forget: you have to see clearly.

If you use a lens with a larger diameter than that of the cornea you may also "indent" the cornea and open some parts of the angle. If the patient does not look straight ahead, the rim of the lens will indent the cornea and some aqueous humor will be displaced. The part of the angle opposite the indentation will get wider. The same effect is possible if you as the examiner tilt the lens some degrees out of the central axis. Unintended indentation may artificially open an angle! One sign of indentation are striae of the cornea, as mentioned above.

2.4 Surroundings

Gonioscopy should be performed in a relatively dark room. Otherwise the consensual pupillary reaction will constrict the pupil of the examined eye. Therefore, a room with a low light level is recommended. You may start with a brighter beam to get an overview of the angle structures. Afterwards reduce the brightness and the size of the slit beam. Use a short (2–3 mm), not too wide (1 mm) and not too bright slit beam. Otherwise ITCs (appositions) cannot be diagnosed correctly, and may be missed. And you would miss the need to perform neodymium:yttrium-aluminum-garnet (Nd:YAG) laser iridotomy. Perform "dark room gonioscopy" in all eyes with a suspicion of angle closure disease and in all eyes in which the van Herick test is suspicious for possible angle closure. In addition, you may probably find hidden signs of other diseases such as neovascularizations or increased pigmentation.

2.5 Tonometry or Gonioscopy: Which First?

Always perform tonometry first. The pressure during gonioscopy may reduce the intraocular pressure artificially. The anesthetic compound in fluorecain eye drops for tonometry will be sufficient to do gonioscopy afterwards.

2.6 Importance of Gonioscopy

Glaucoma is not the only pathology that should point you towards examining the chamber angle by gonioscopy. There are many other pathologies changing the configuration of parts of the angle, such as tumors that will never lead to glaucoma. A foreign body may be hidden behind the peripheral cornea and the patient only remembers a "second of pain", has no blurred vision and no red eye (Figs. 2.12 and 2.13).

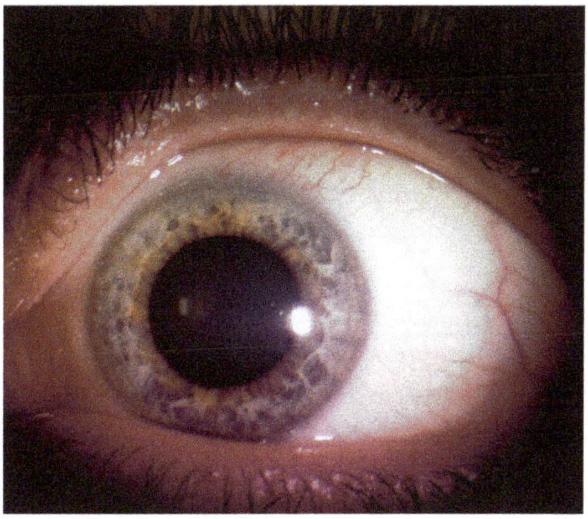

Fig. 2.12 Right eye after a penetrating injury. The patient was not aware that a foreign body had entered his eye. There is only a low grade conjunctival redness superiorly and there are no signs of an intraocular foreign body on slit lamp examination

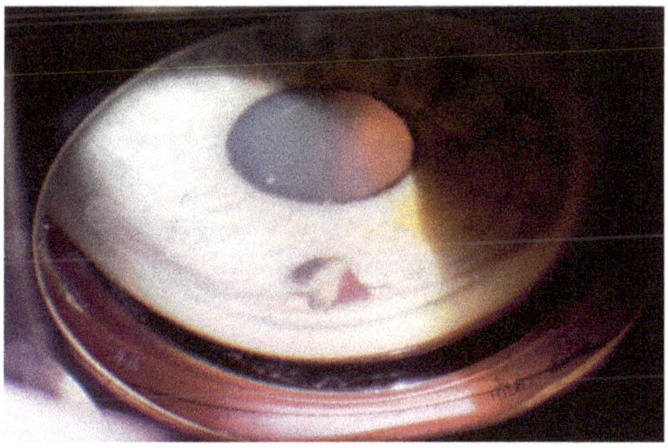

Fig. 2.13 Same eye as shown in Fig. 2.12. Gonioscopy revealed an encapsulated foreign body with a peripheral coloboma at 12 o'clock. The foreign body was extracted using a magnet

Bibliography

Alward WL, Longmuir RA (2008) Color atlas of gonioscopy, 2nd edn. American Academy of Ophthalmology, San Francisco

Becker SC, Grüning HD (1976) Gonioskopie. Lehrbuch und Atlas mit stereoskopischen Bildern. Schattauer, Stuttgart

Forbes M (1966) Gonioscopy with corneal indentation. Arch Ophthalmol 76:488–492

Barkana Y, Dorairaj SK, Gerber Y, Liebmann JM, Ritch R (2007) Agreement between gonioscopy and ultrasound biomicroscopy in detecting iridotrabecular apposition. Arch Ophthalmol 125:1331–1335

Palmberg P (2007) Shedding light on gonioscopy (editorial). Arch Ophthalmol 125:1417–1418

Schirmer KE (1967) Gonioscopy and artefacts. Br J Ophthalmol 51:50–53

European Glaucoma Society (2008) Terminology and guidelines for glaucoma, 3rd edn. Dogma, Savona

Walland MJ, Ravi T (2010) So what's our angle on this? (editorial). Clin Exp Ophthalmol 38:743–744

Anatomical Structures of the Chamber Angle

3

Any angle is framed by two parts: in the eye's anterior chamber angle one side is the iris, the other side is the end (or beginning) of the cornea, the corneoscleral trabeculum (with Schlemm's canal partially behind), part of the sclera and part of the ciliary muscle. In fact, it is not a real geometrical angle; it is a concave recess formed by the structures described below.

A histological section of the chamber angle gives a wonderful overview of the structures involved (Fig. 3.1). Take a few minutes and remember what you have learned in anatomy and histology. The schematic drawing shown in Fig. 3.2 reduces the visual information to its important elements.

You can start your analysis from the cornea or from the iris. You can get good results either way.

We start our description of the several structures or "landmarks" of the chamber angle in detail in an anterior (i.e. the cornea) to posterior direction (Fig. 3.3).

3.1 Schwalbe's Line or Ring

- *Definition*: It is a condensation of collagen tissue and highlights the end or beginning of Descemet's membrane (Fig. 3.4). Schwalbe's line is better called Schwalbe's ring, because it runs circumferentially as a ring and has no start point or end point.
- *Is it easy to find?* Not in eyes with no, little or not very much pigment. It is translucent and slightly more white than the close anterior trabeculum. *Tip*: Use the "corneal wedge" technique: the very slim and oblique beam of the slit lamp is separated into an exterior part (corneal epithelium) and an interior part (corneal endothelium) of the transparent cornea and crosses the inner slit beam of the non-transparent scleral tissue (trabecular meshwork). This crossing defines Schwalbe's ring (Fig. 3.5). This technique is very useful in eyes with (almost) no pigmentation or very dense pigmentation of the angle.

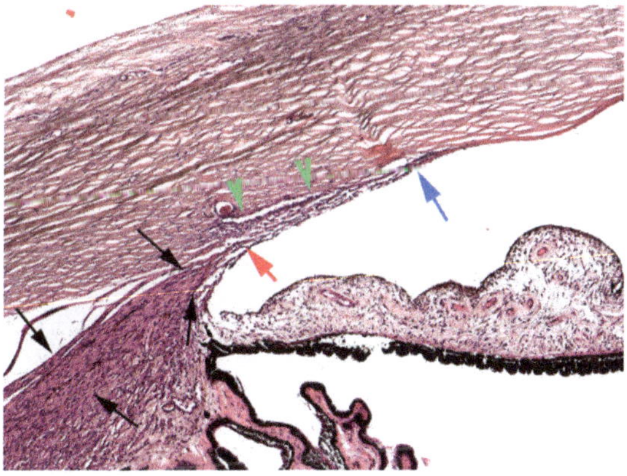

Fig. 3.1 Histological section of a chamber angle (Masson trichrome). The chamber angle of a human eye is not a pointed angle; it is a recess made up of Schwalbe's ring (*blue arrow*), the trabecular meshwork (*between blue and red arrows*), the scleral spur (*red arrow*), the anterior ciliary muscle and the iris. The longitudinal parts of the ciliary muscle insert at the scleral spur (*between the black arrows*). *Green arrows* external wall of Schlemm's canal (courtesy R. Kleinert)

C. Faschinger, A. Hommer, *Gonioscopy*,
DOI 10.1007/978-3-642-28610-0_3, © Springer-Verlag Berlin Heidelberg 2012

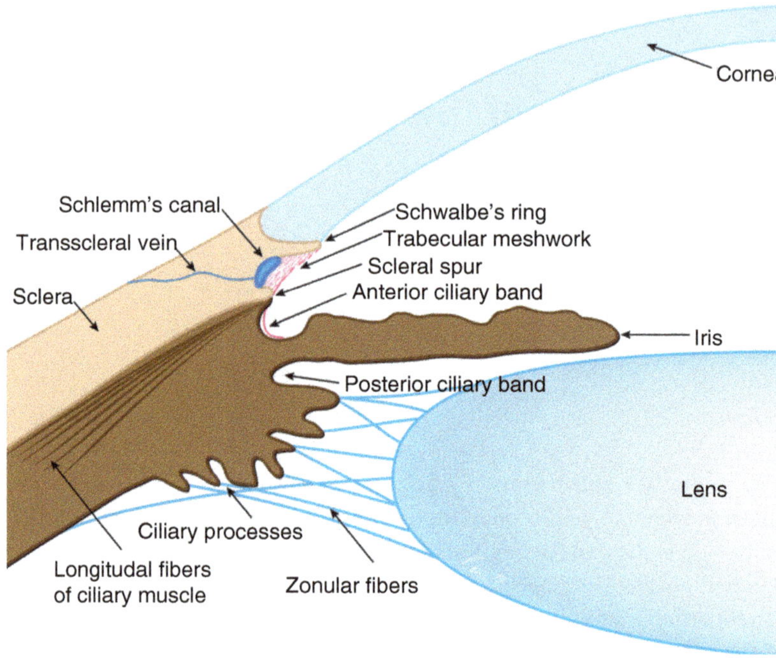

Fig. 3.2 Schematic drawing of the chamber angle with all important structures. This schema is used throughout the book

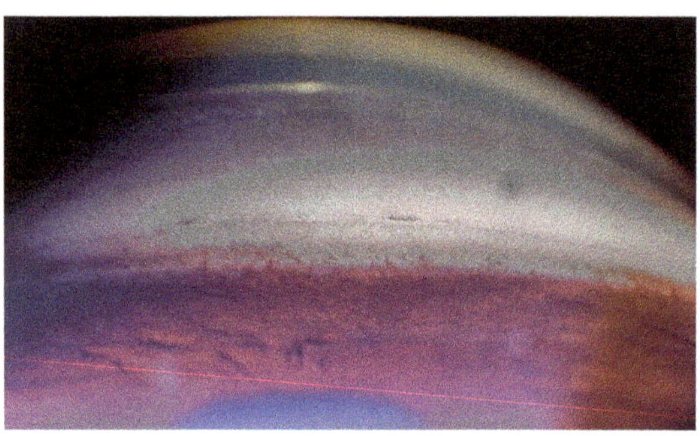

Fig. 3.3 All structures of a normal chamber angle

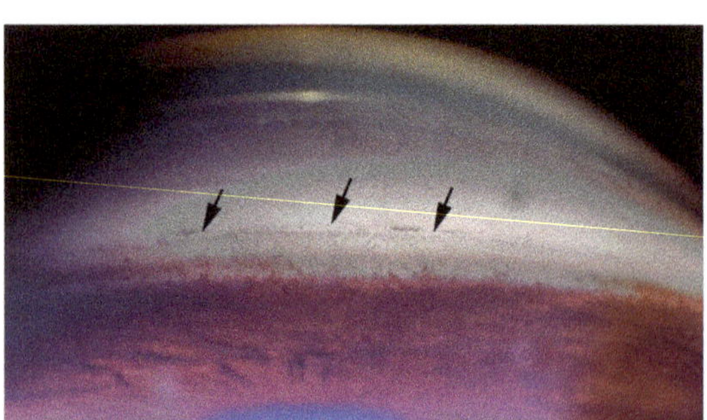

Fig. 3.4 Schwalbe's ring (*black arrows*) as white thin thickening at the beginning of Descemet's membrane between the cornea and the nonfunctional part of the trabecular meshwork

- *Is it important?*
  - Yes, because normal vessels and normal tissue will not pass it. Pathological vessels (in neovascularization) and pathological tissue (peripheral anterior synechiae, PAS) may pass Schwalbe's ring up to the cornea and anteriorly.
- *Who is it named after?* Gustav Schwalbe, German anatomist, 1844–1910. Jean Descemet, French anatomist, 1732–1810.
- *Does it show variations?* Yes, Schwalbe's ring may be prominent with the appearance of a ledge, and is then called "embryotoxon posterius". Greek *toxon* means "bow", because in most eyes only a part (nasal and/or temporal) of Schwalbe's ring is prominent and therefore looks like a bow. All these eyes have no increased risk of glaucoma. You may see this prominent white ring even with the slit lamp (Fig. 3.6).

3.2 Trabecular Meshwork

- *Definition*: Many collagen fibers: (Latin *trabs* = bar) are coated with endothelium and form a specific meshwork. There is a non-functional

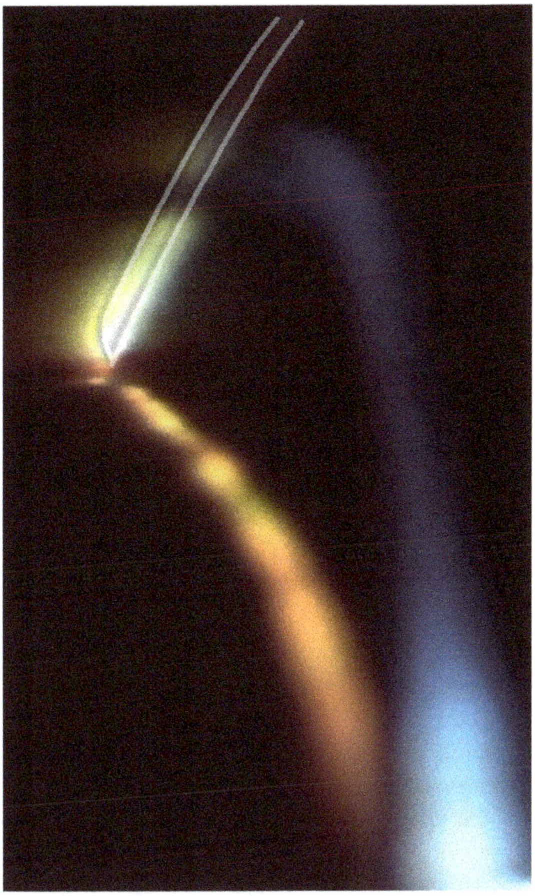

Fig. 3.5 Schwalbe's ring can also be identified by the "corneal wedge". The slit beam is reflected by the anterior, external surface of the cornea and the posterior, internal surface of the cornea (artificially highlighted). Where these two reflections merge and cross the inner reflex of the angle, there is Schwalbe's ring

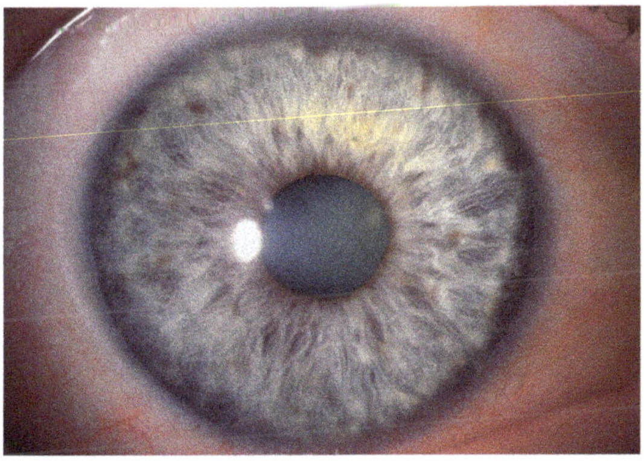

Fig. 3.6 The thickened Schwalbe's ring called embryotoxon posterius is easily recognized temporally and nasally

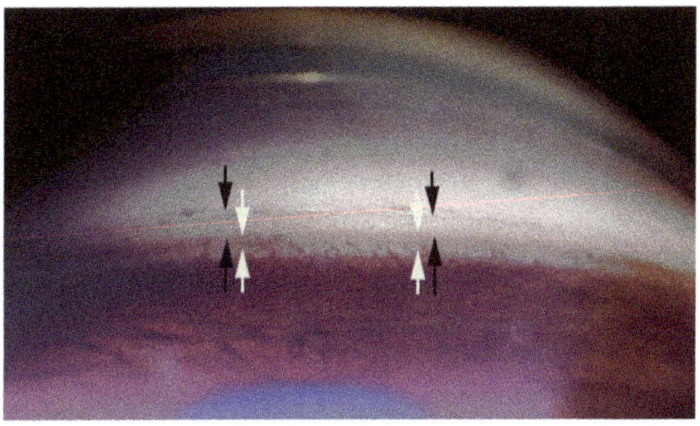

Fig. 3.7 Nonfunctional trabecular meshwork (*between the black arrows*) is paler than the functional part of the trabecular meshwork (*between the white arrows*) and both are between Schwalbe's ring and the scleral spur. Pigmentation grade +2 (Scheie)

and a functional part (Fig. 3.7). The *non-functional* part has (almost) no outflow function due to lack of a canal behind it. In front of Schlemm's canal is the *functional part* for the aqueous humor outflow, which controls the flow resistance (trabecular facility) to maintain equilibrium between production and outflow. It is also called the posterior trabecular meshwork. The trabeculum has a width of approximately 600 μm and consists of three layers:

- Uveoscleral trabeculum with large pores (25 μm) running from Schwalbe's line to the ciliary muscle. (Macrophages have a diameter of 20–30 μm.)
- Corneoscleral trabeculum with smaller pores (2–12 μm) running from Schwalbe's line to the scleral spur. (Erythrocytes have a diameter of 7.5 μm, leukocytes 13 μm.)
- Juxtacanalicular or cribriform trabeculum (Latin *cribrum* = strainer) forms the inner wall of Schlemm's canal. There are no openings to the canal. Vesicles of the aqueous humor are transported through the endothelial cells and the connective tissue. Due to changes of the extracellular matrix and the cells it is *the* region for increased resistance in primary open-angle glaucoma (OAG). The outflow is pressure-dependent. Of the aqueous humor, 70–90% passes through this way, if the IOP is higher than the pressure in the episcleral veins.

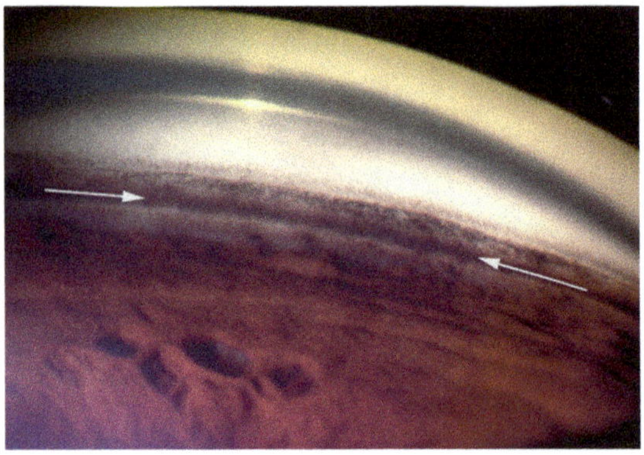

Fig. 3.8 Black pigment grade +4 of the functional trabecular meshwork (*arrows*) in an eye with pigmentary glaucoma. The nonfunctional trabecular meshwork is also pigmented

- *Is it easy to find?* Yes, when there is pigment. Not so easy in children or in eyes with no pigment.
- *Is it important?*
  - Yes, for surgical procedures targeting exactly this tissue (surgery with the goniotomy knife, surgery with the excimer laser or with a Trabectome, implantation of stents such as the iStent).
  - Yes, for laser therapy. In particular, in argon laser trabeculoplasty, the spots have to be located as exactly as possible between the nonfunctional and the functional part.
  - Yes, if it is covered by iris tissue (reversible apposition or irreversible synechia); then called angle closure. The quality of the trabecular meshwork cells will deteriorate after a certain period of appositional closure.
- *Grade the amount of pigment*: Scheie suggested a system of grading (0 none, +1 trace, +2 mild, +3 moderate, +4 severe; Fig. 3.8). Granular pigment, especially in the inferior part of the angle due to gravitation and convection currents, increases with age, in diabetes, after trauma or Nd:YAG iridotomy or angle-closure attack or uveitis, in pseudoexfoliation syndrome/glaucoma ("pepper and salt", variegated; "pepper" is the blackish pigment, and "salt" is the elastin material; irregular pigmentation) or in pigmentary dispersion syndrome/glaucoma ("more brown pepper", homogeneous). Grade the amount of pigmentation of the posterior trabecular meshwork at the 12 o'clock position!
- The pattern of pigment granule deposition may vary depending on the cause: after the release of a previous angle closure (iridotrabecular contact, ITC) in angle closure, the pigment of the iris leaves a distinct geographic blotch on the trabecular meshwork. The granules have a fluffy and tufted appearance without a gravitational distribution.
- *Note*: the cells of the trabecular meshwork are active cells! They may contract or relax due to the action of actin filaments.

3.3 Schlemm's Canal

- *Definition*: A canal with a lumen of 121 ± 45 μm runs circumferentially between the cornea and the sclera draining the aqueous humor via collector vessels to the episcleral and conjunctival veins.
- *Is it easy to find?* Schlemm's canal is only visible when filled with blood. This might happen in hypotonia bulbi, during resorption of hyphema or in several diseases involving increased episcleral venous pressure, a fistula of the carotis in the sinus cavernosus or in Sturge-Weber syndrome. If you apply pressure to the limbal sclera with the edge of the contact lens during examination, Schlemm's canal might fill with some blood from the episcleral veins.
- *Who is it named after?* Friedrich Schlemm, 1795–1858, found the blood-filled canal in hanged persons. Formerly it was called "sinus venosus sclerae".
- *Important?*
  - Yes, 75–90% of the aqueous humor passes this way through the trabecular meshwork to Schlemm's canal (conventional outflow, pressure-dependent, IOP higher than pressure in the episcleral veins).
  - Yes, for surgical procedures targeting exactly this canal (canaloplasty, trabeculotomy, viscocanalostomy, implants into the canal).

3.4 Scleral Spur

- *Definition*: Ridge of collagen tissue of the sclera (Fig. 3.9).
- *Is it easy to find?* Yes, because it is white and bright. It is *the* most important landmark. It might be invisible due to the forward bowing of the iris. Then an angle closure is possible. If the scleral spur is visible, an angle closure is almost excludable.
- *Is it important?*
  - Yes, for the differential diagnosis between open-angle and angle-closure glaucoma.
  - Yes. It is the end of the corneoscleral trabeculum. Fibers of the longitudinal part of the ciliary muscle (Brücke's muscle) insert here and may open the trabeculum when the muscle contracts (especially by the action of cholinergic agents such as pilocarpine). A side effect is anterior rotation and thickening of the ciliary body.
- *Does it show variations?* Sometimes the scleral spur is covered by uveal tissue as small, sharp-ended processes from the iris root running up to the trabeculum (Fig. 3.10) These are called *iris processes*. They are probably evolutionary remnants (*ligamentum pectinatum*; Latin *pectin*=comb) or represent incomplete cleavage during maturation of the angle. They are found in one-third of brown eyes in younger individuals, but they have no pathological consequences and are not associated with a higher risk of development of glaucoma except when they are numerous and combined with anterior synechiae (AS; Fig. 3.11), in which case 50% will develop glaucoma in late childhood or early adulthood (Rieger anomaly). Spaeth classified them as pilaster-like fibers (short U fibers), fibers up to the scleral spur or posterior trabecular meshwork (V fibers), and fibers reaching Schwalbe's ring (W fibers). They gradually diminish with age.

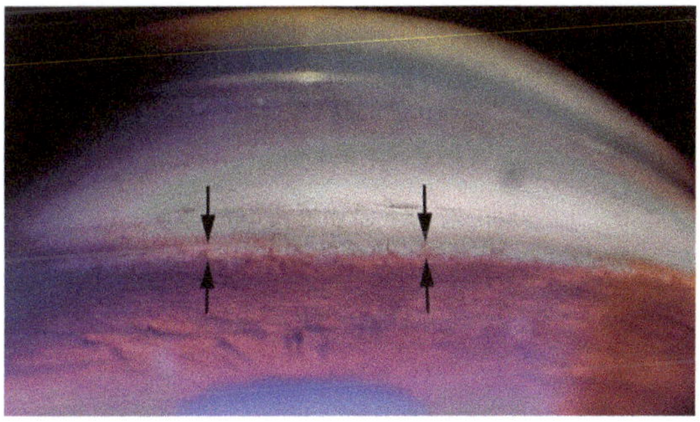

Fig. 3.9 Bright white scleral spur as a thickening of the sclera between the functional part of the trabecular meshwork and the anterior ciliary band (*between the arrows*)

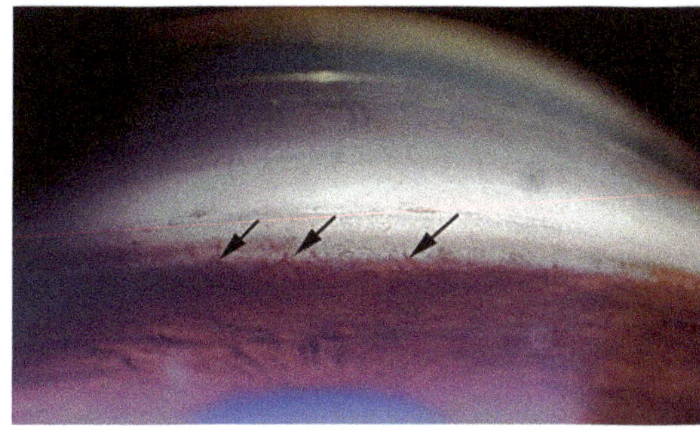

Fig. 3.10 Iris processes as small, sharp-ending processes running from the iris root up to the trabeculum (*arrows*). They have no pathological consequences in relation to glaucoma

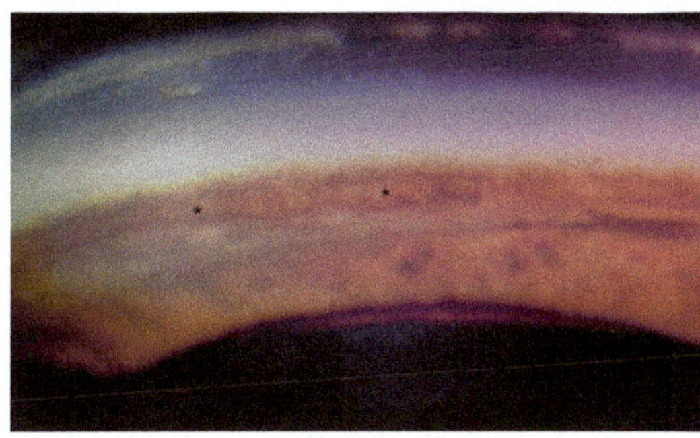

Fig. 3.11 Chamber angle with very dense iris processus increasing the IOP (*asterisks* show the region where the scleral spur might be expected)

3.5 Anterior Ciliary Muscle Band

- *Definition*: Visible part of the longitudinal fibers of the ciliary muscle (Brücke's muscle) (Fig. 3.12).
- *Is it easy to find?* Yes, as light-brown greyish tissue in open angles. It is wide in eyes with deep angles as in high myopia, after trauma with subluxation of the lens, and in aphakia

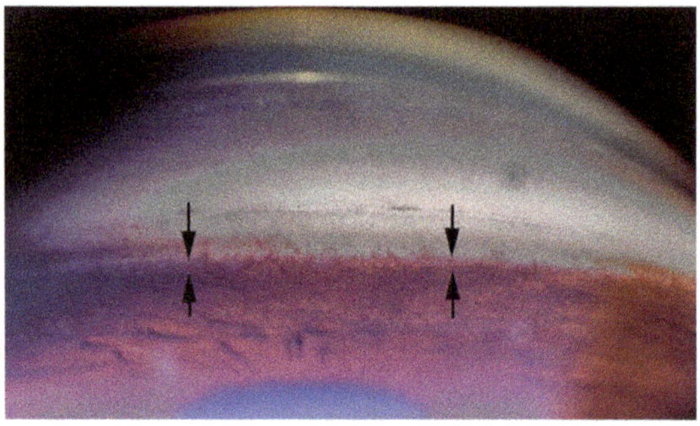

Fig. 3.12 Dark-brown anterior ciliary band (*between the arrows*) reaching from the scleral spur to the insertion of the iris

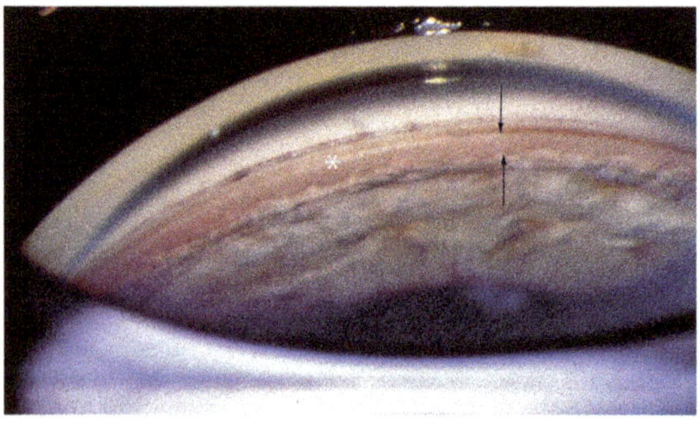

Fig. 3.13 Deep anterior chamber and wide-open chamber angle with a very broad anterior ciliary band (*between the arrows*; *asterisk* scleral spur). Trabecular meshwork pigmentation grade +2 to +3; eye with high myopia

(Fig. 3.13). It is narrow or missing in very short eyes (hyperopia) and in anterior insertion of the iris.

- *Is it important?*
  - Yes. If visible an angle closure can be ruled out.
  - Yes. Ten to twenty five percent of the aqueous humor passes through the ciliary band to the suprachoroidal space (nonconventional outflow, increased mainly by prostaglandin analogues). If the IOP is less than the episcleral venous pressure, all aqueous humor passes through the ciliary band (Fig. 3.14).

3.6 Iris Root and Iris

- *Definition*: Connective tissue of two leaves (anterior stromal layer with chromatophores and posterior pigmented layer with muscles) forming the aperture called the pupil. Normally there are vessels in the iris stroma running circumferentially or radially.
- *Is it easy to find?* Yes.
- *Is it important?* Yes. It allows different configurations of angles. The peripheral part,

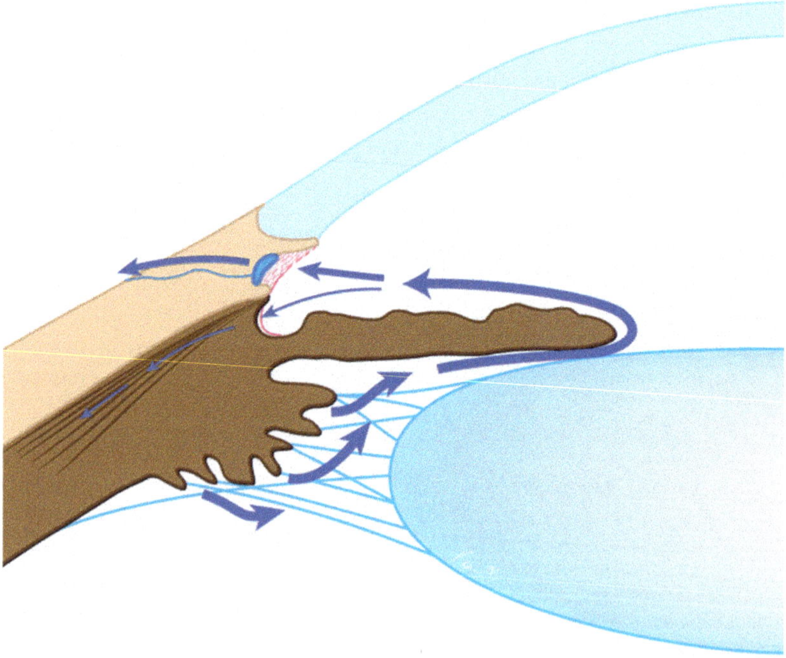

Fig. 3.14 Aqueous humor leaves the eye in two ways: a pressure-dependent way via the trabecular meshwork, Schlemm's canal, intrascleral vessels and episcleral veins, and a non-pressure-dependent way via the ciliary muscle, suprachoroidal space and transscleral vessels to the veins

or final roll, named after Fuchs, is thinner than the central part with the sphincter, and therefore forward bowing occurs leading to ITC/apposition or PAS. Beyond the final roll is the angle recess.

- *Does it show variations?*
  - *"Insertion" of the iris*: Insertion is defined as the point of the iris where it *visually* "inserts". This may be on the ciliary body, but also upwards on the corneal endothelium.
  - Normally the insertion of the iris is deep (Fig. 3.15d) posterior to the (anterior) ciliary band or is extremely deep (Fig. 3.15e) at the ciliary body. Sometimes, the insertion is at the scleral spur (Fig. 3.15c; this is seen particularly in young individuals), behind Schwalbe's ring (Fig. 3.15b) or anterior (Fig. 3.15a) to the trabecular meshwork. Insertion behind Schwalbe's ring (Fig. 3.15b) also means between Schwalbe's ring and the scleral spur. Figure 3.15a, b shows high "insertions" which may be associated with developmental or secondary glaucoma.
  - *Configuration of the peripheral iris*: Normally the *peripheral* iris is flat or regular (f or R configuration; Fig. 3.16). In eyes with pigment dispersion syndrome/glaucoma, or in eyes with subluxation of the lens, the peripheral iris is bowed backward (c for concave configuration); this is also called the queer (Q) configuration. In angle closure or plateau-iris configuration the peripheral iris is bowed forward (convex); this is called the steep configuration (S or b for bowing forward and p for plateau configuration; Fig. 3.16).
- *Pathology*: There are two important terms (that should not to be confused with iris processus):
  - *ITC or apposition* (Figs. 3.17 and 3.18): The narrowest part of the angle is between the peripheral iris roll (Fuchs) on one side and the trabecular meshwork and Schwalbe's ring on the opposite side. In this area both tissues may come into contact. Apposition is fully reversible, and does not cause symptoms. Reasons for apposition include dilation of the pupil in occludable angles, "intermittent" angle closure with pupillary block, and forward bowing of the peripheral iris.
  - *Synechiae*: Tissue of the iris that remains strongly in contact with the trabeculum or Schwalbe's ring is called PAS (Fig. 3.19). In exact anatomical terms it is a "goniosynechia" when the iris is in contact with parts of the chamber angle, and it is an "anterior synechia" (Fig. 3.19c, d) when the iris is in contact with the cornea beyond the chamber angle.
  - *Important*: Differentiation between an ITC/apposition and a synechia is only possible by indentation gonioscopy.
  - In contrast to appositions, a PAS is not reversible, except by surgery (goniosynechialysis). Symptoms due to synechiae are rare. The reasons for PAS are diverse: after penetrating injuries, after inflammation, in chronic angle closure, pushing the iris–lens diaphragm anteriorly (e.g. gas after vitreoretinal surgery), or pulling it anteriorly (fibrovascular tissue in neovascularizations, in iridocorneal-endothelial syndromes), or after improper argon-laser trabeculoplasty (too close to the ciliary band).
- *What else?* Watch the surface of the iris: is there dotted pigment (in pigment dispersion syndrome/glaucoma, pseudoexfoliation syndrome/glaucoma; Fig. 3.20)? Is the iris partially atrophic (after herpes zoster, after acute angle-closure attack), split (iridoschisis; Fig. 3.21) or twisted (after acute angle-closure attack) (Fig. 3.22). Is the stromal layer noticeably thin such that the vessels are very easily detectable (Fuchs uveitis)? Are there vessels in a randomized pattern (neovascularization, new vessels on the surface of the iris; Fig. 3.23)? On transillumination of the iris are there peripheral defects of the pigmented layer (pigment dispersion syndrome/glaucoma) or are they located in the middle or center (after herpes). *And*: do not forget to check the color of both irises (heterochromia, in Fuchs uveitis; Fig. 3.24).

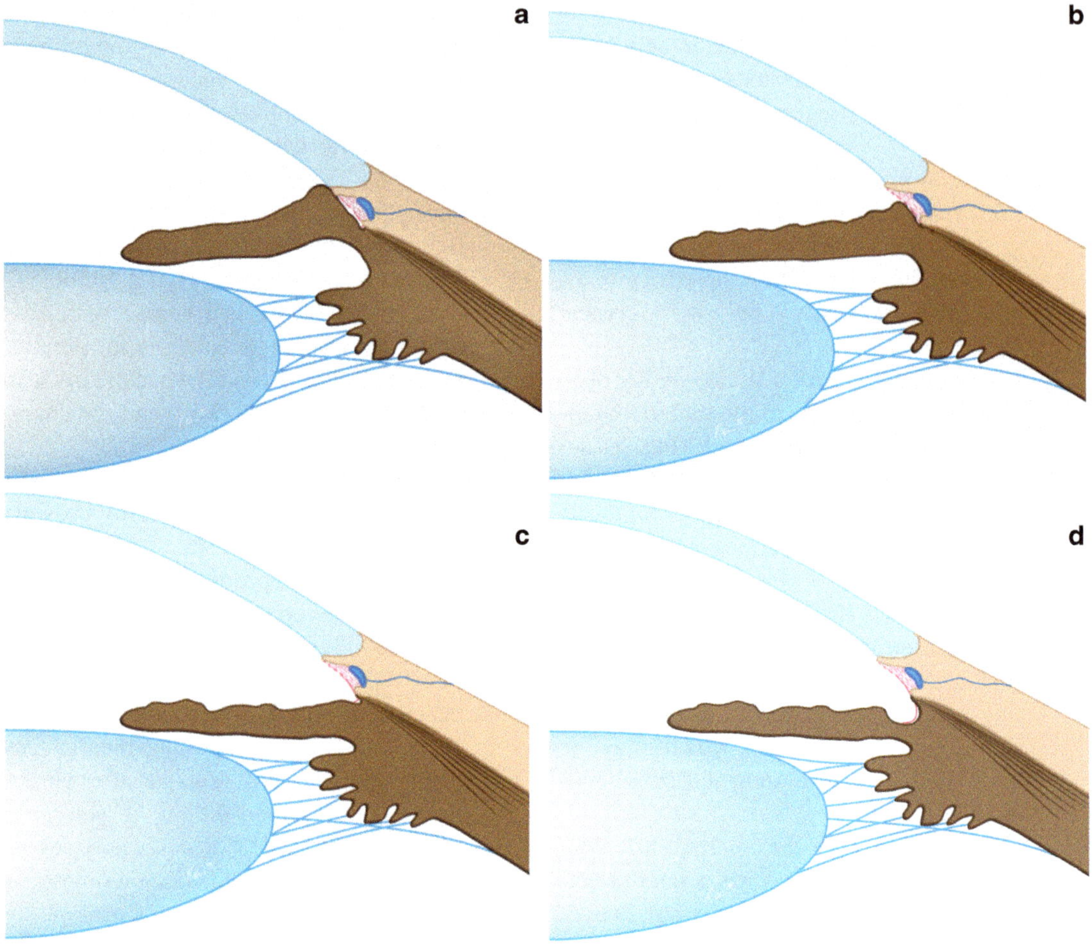

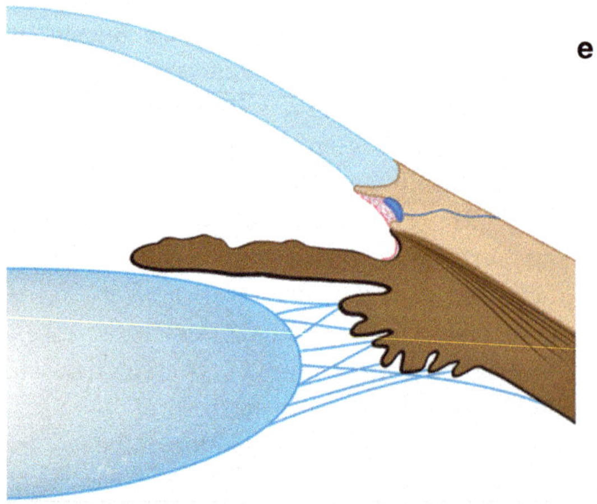

a	Anterior to trabecular meshwork
b	Behind Schwalbe´s ring or between Schwalbe´s ring and scleral spur
c	At scleral spur
d	Deep
e	Extremely deep

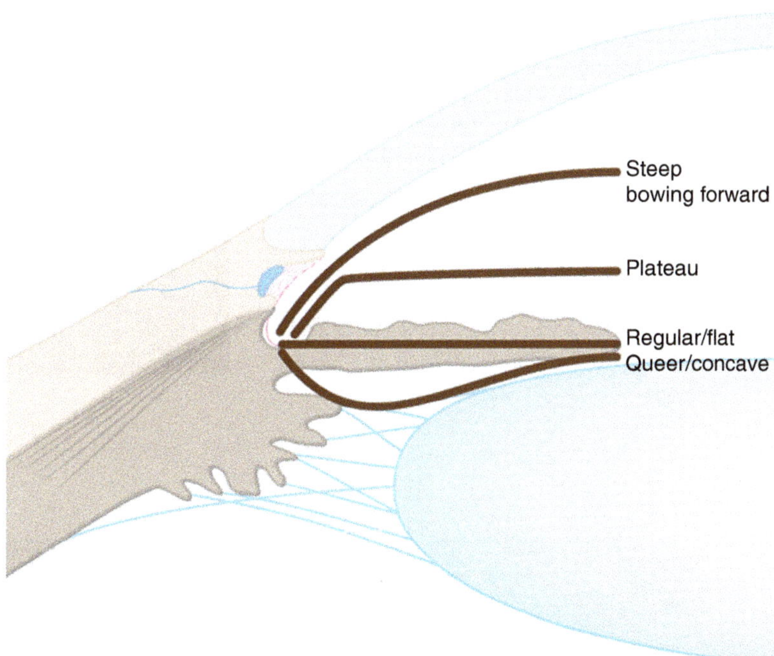

Fig. 3.16 Four possible configurations of the iris: steep or bowed forward (S or b), plateau-like (p), regular or flat (R or f) and queer (Q) or concave (c)

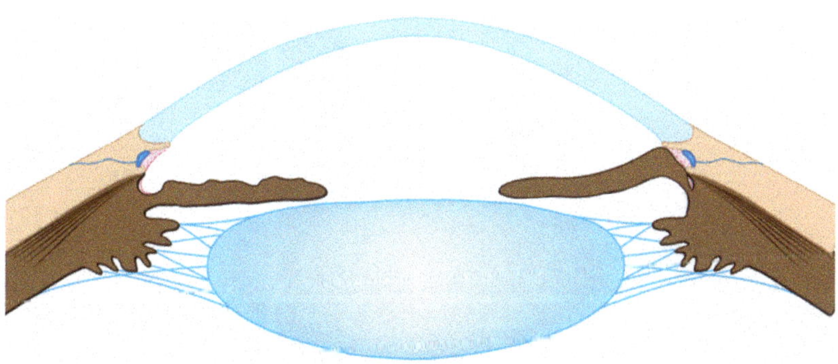

Fig. 3.17 The chamber angle on the *left* side is wide open (there is a distance between the trabecular meshwork and the peripheral iris), in contrast to the *right* side, where the chamber angle is closed. The iris is in contact with the trabecular meshwork. Whether this closure is a contact or a synechia can only be determined by indentation gonioscopy

Fig. 3.15 (**a**) The iris is in contact with the cornea anterior to Schwalbe's ring (e.g. in secondary glaucoma due to pathological growth of the endothelial cells in iridocorneal-endothelial syndrome). (**b**) The iris is in contact with the trabecular meshwork between Schwalbe's ring and the scleral spur (e.g. in secondary angle closure due to neovascularizations). (**c**) The iris is in contact with the anterior ciliary band close to the scleral spur, which is visible (e.g. it is uncommon, but is seen in young individuals). (**d**) The iris inserts at the ciliary body. This is the most frequent insertion. (**e**) The insertion of the iris is very deep at the ciliary body (e.g. in highly myopic eyes)

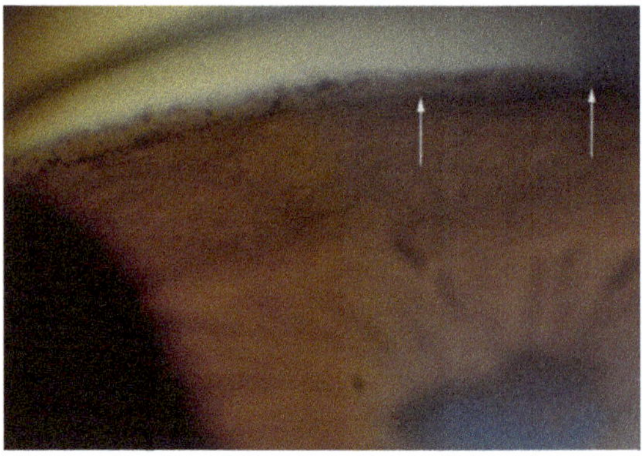

Fig. 3.18 ITC or peripheral anterior synechia (differentiation only by indentation gonioscopy). Only the nonfunctional part of the trabecular meshwork and some clotted pigment is visible, besides a small part of the functional trabecular meshwork (*between the arrows*)

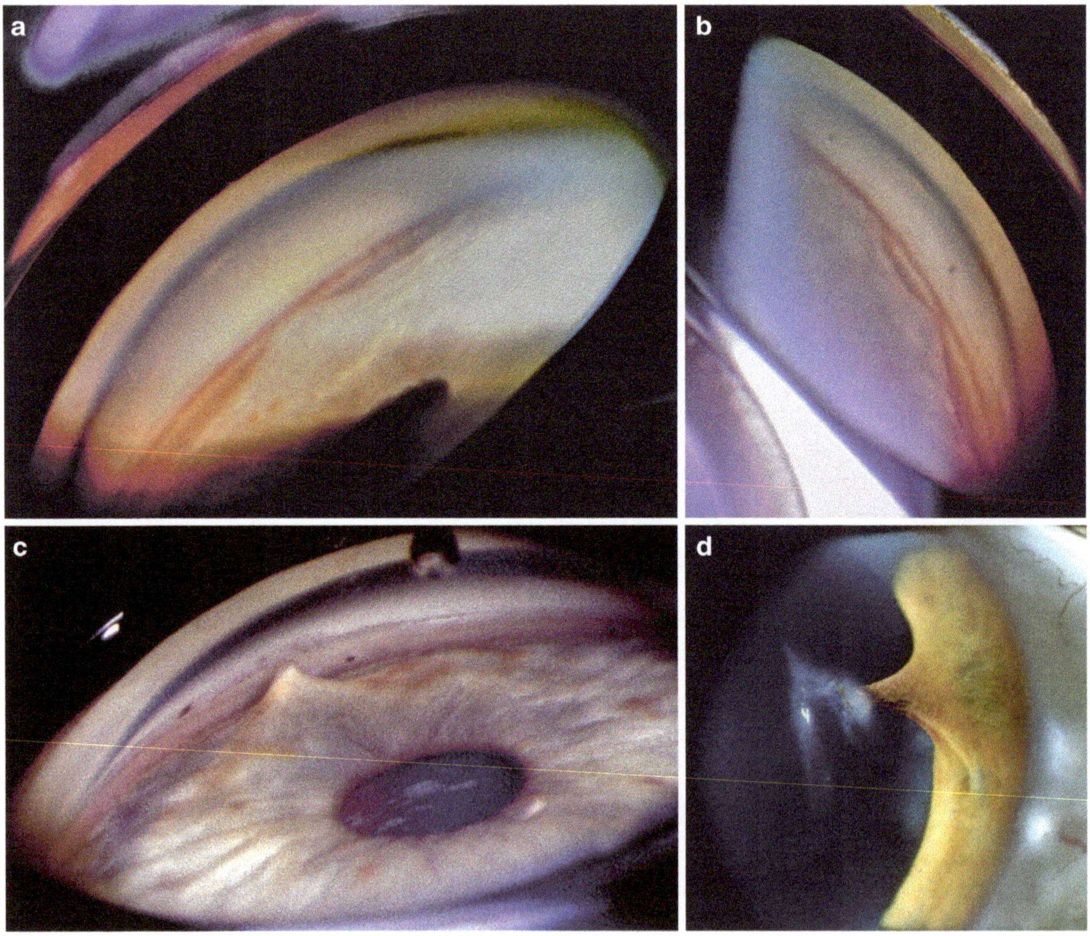

Fig. 3.19 (**a**) Peripheral anterior synechiae with a broad base, and a triangular shape. The major part of the chamber angle is wide open; the pigmented trabecular meshwork, the scleral spur and the anterior ciliary band are easily detectable. (**b**) Peripheral anterior synechia runs from the iris to Schwalbe's ring. (**c**, **d**) An anterior synechia runs from the iris up to the cornea due to a penetrating injury of the eyeball

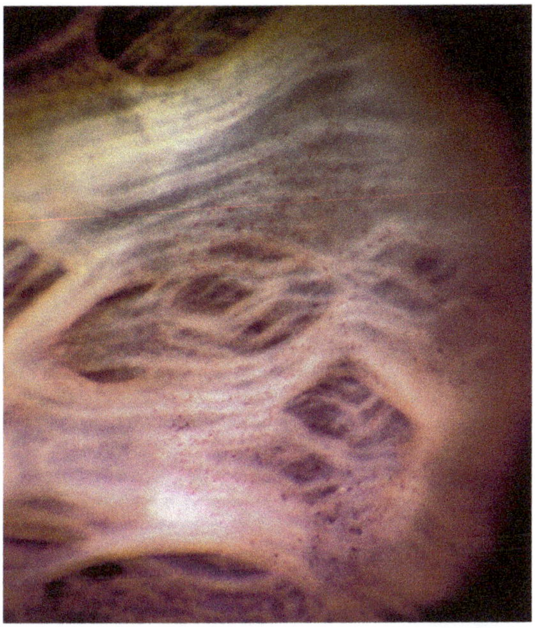

Fig. 3.20 Dotted pigment granules on the surface of the iris in an eye with pigmentary glaucoma

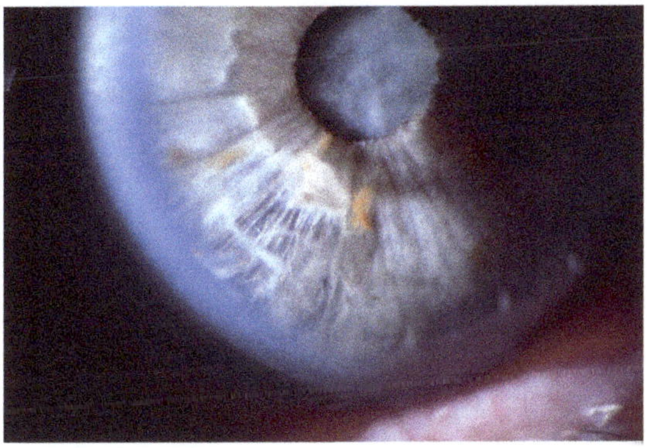

Fig. 3.21 Splitting of the anterior layer of the iris, called iridoschisis, mostly in the inferior parts

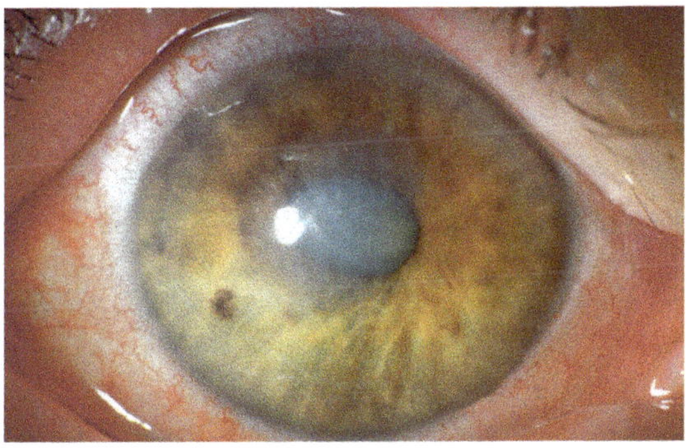

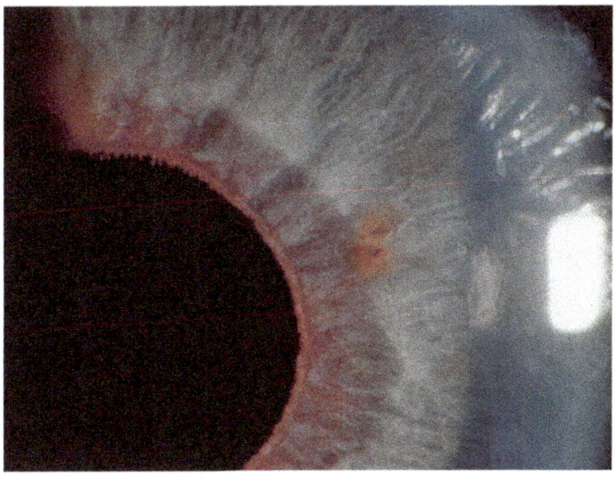

Fig. 3.23 Thin, newly formed vessels in a random pattern in an eye 6 months after central venous occlusion

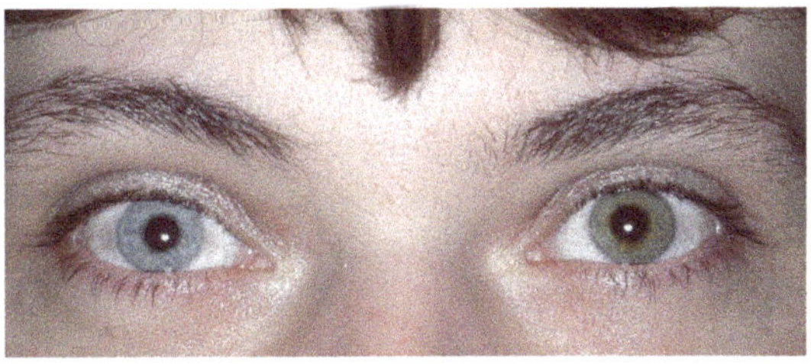

Fig. 3.24 Irises of different color in Fuchs heterochromic uveitis. The right eye is the eye with the disease

3.7 Posterior Ciliary Muscle Band, Ciliary Sulcus

- *Definition*: Space between the posterior part of the iris and the anterior parts of the ciliary body processes and the circular parts (Müller's muscle) of the ciliary muscle.
- *Is it easy to find?* It is usually invisible, but is visible in eyes with aniridia or iridodialysis, in eyes with widely dilated pupils, or when the ciliary body is rotated anteriorly (in plateau-iris configuration).
- *Is it important?* In former days the loops of intraocular lenses where positioned in the ciliary sulcus. Since the invention of the circular anterior capsulorhexis, the capsular bag is in

Fig. 3.22 Twisted stromal fibers of the anterior layer of the iris after an acute angle-closure attack. The central cornea is still edematous

its proper physiological place. Nowadays, the loops of add-on intraocular lenses to correct postoperative refractive errors or implantable contact plate-haptic lenses are placed in the ciliary sulcus.

- *Does it show variations?* In eyes with plateau-iris configurations the ciliary sulcus may be very narrow or even absent. Then Nd:YAG laser iridotomy will not help, because the iris has no space to fall backwards. These eyes need an additional argon-laser peripheral iridoplasty.

3.8 Blood Vessels

The blood vessels run from the greater circle of the iris (circulus arteriosus iridis major) circumferentially in the angle or radially towards the pupil. Pathological vessels extend to Schwalbe's ring or further anteriorly, are thinner and of randomized patterns.

Do they show variations? In eyes with Fuchs' uveitis, blood will spontaneously flush out of the vessels of the chamber angle if the IOP is very low or zero, i.e. when a paracentesis is done in cataract or glaucoma surgery. This is called the Amsler-Verrey sign.

3.9 Sampaolesi's Line

- *Definition*: Sampaolesi's line is a pigmented line and is mostly found only in the inferior part of the chamber angle, anterior to Schwalbe's ring in some eyes (Figs. 3.25 and 3.26).
- *Is it easy to find?* Yes, because it is pigmented and close to the whitish Schwalbe's ring. Sometimes it is slightly undulating and not straight.
- *Is it important?* Most eyes with a Sampaolesi's line have pigment dispersion syndrome/glaucoma or a pseudoexfoliation syndrome/glaucoma, but not all. It is not pathognomonic for a particular disease.
- *Who is it named after?* Roberto Sampaolesi, ophthalmologist, of Buenos Aires, Argentina.

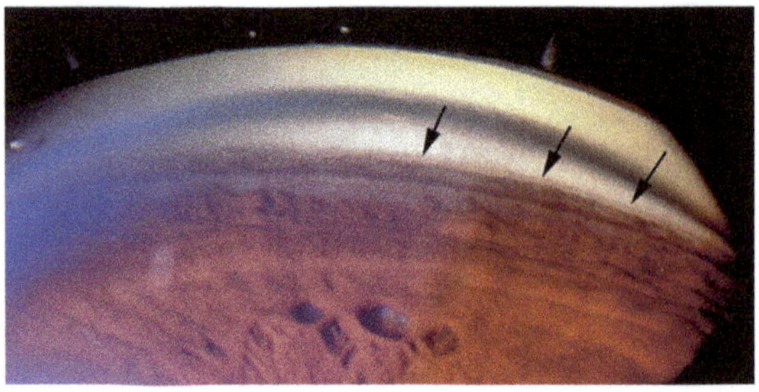

Fig. 3.25 Pigmented Sampaolesi's line (*arrows*) anterior to a thin white Schwalbe's ring in an eye with pigment glaucoma. Note the broad anterior ciliary band, the heavily pigmented functional (grade +4) and even the pigmented nonfunctional trabecular meshwork between the scleral spur and Schwalbe's ring

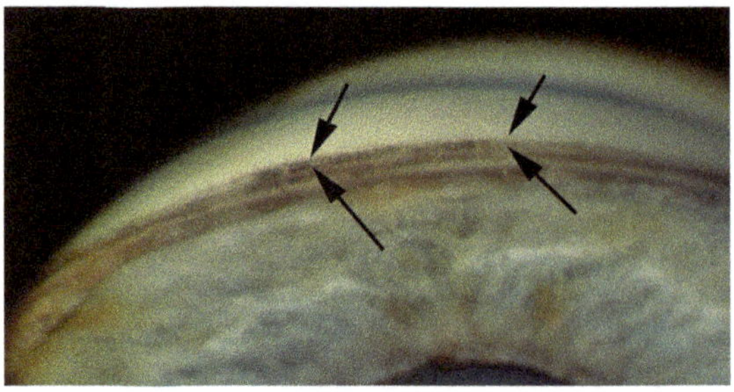

Fig. 3.26 Pigmented Sampaolesi's line (*between the arrows*) in an eye with pseudoexfoliation glaucoma. The pigmentation of the chamber angle is less pronounced as in an eye with pigmentary glaucoma

- *Differential diagnosis*: Be careful not to confuse it with spotted pigment granules after Nd:YAG laser iridotomy, which are also found in the inferior part of the chamber angle. An iridotomy releases a large amount of iris pigment. Very undulated pigmented lines may have developed after the release of iridotrabecular adhesions in acute angle-closure disease.

3.10 Lens

The position of the lens (anterior, regular or posterior) as well as the configuration due to its thickness (thicker in advanced cataract) have to be taken into account. Thick or anteriorly displaced lenses may induce closure of the angle by causing a pupillary block.

3.11 Cornea

In eyes with pseudoexfoliation syndrome/glaucoma the endothelium of the cornea shows spot-like pigment and/or whitish material. In eyes with pigment dispersion syndrome/glaucoma, vertical spindle-like deposits of pigment reach from 6 to 12 o'clock (Krukenberg). Eyes with anterior uveitis show different amounts of white cells on the endothelium. Horizontal and circumferential tears of Descemet's membrane are typical of buphthalmus.

3.12 Decision Tree

IOP increase and/or typical changes of the disc/RNFL and/or typical glaucomatous visual field defects

Regular gonioscopy:

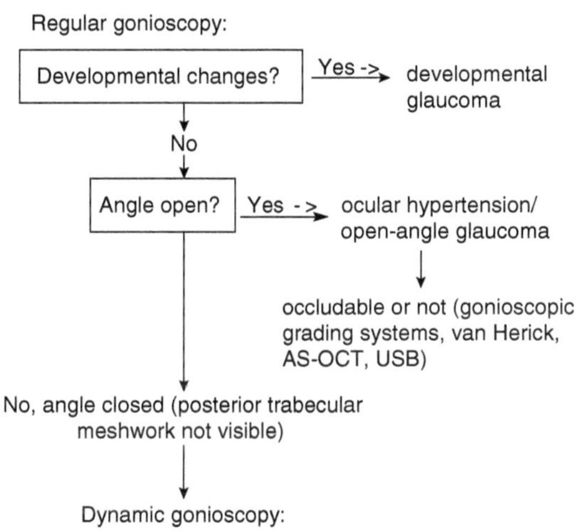

Dynamic gonioscopy:

- Apposition, ITC: primary angle-closure suspect, if IOP <21(PACS)
- Apposition, ITC, synechiae: primary angle-closure, if IOP >21, but visual field and disc/RNFL normal (PAC)
- Apposition, ITC, synechiae: primary angle-closure glaucoma, if IOD >21 and changes in visual field and/or disc/RNFL (PACG)
- Hardly no change in configuration of chamber angle: thick lens
- Double hump: plateau iris configuration

Bibliography

Alward WL, Longmuir RA (2008) Color atlas of gonioscopy, 2nd edn. American Academy of Ophthalmology, San Francisco

Duke-Elder S, Wybar KC (1961) Anterior chamber. In: Duke-Elder S (ed) System of ophthalmology, vol II, The anatomy of the visual system. Kimpton, London

European Glaucoma Society (2008) Terminology and guidelines for glaucoma, 3rd edn. Dogma, Savona

Foster PJ, Gazzard GA, Garway-Heath T, Ritch R (2006) Pattern of trabecular surface pigment deposition in primary angle closure. Arch Ophthalmol 124:1062

Salmon JF (2009) Gonioscopy. In: Shaarawy TM, Sherwood MB, Hitchings RA, Crowstone JG (eds) Glaucoma, vol 1, Medical diagnosis & therapy. Saunders Elsevier, Philadelphia

Wiederholt M (1998) Direct involvement of trabecular meshwork in the regulation of aqueous humour outflow. Curr Opin Ophthalmol 9(2):46–49

Development of the Chamber Angle and Developmental Disorders

4

After gastrulation – that is the formation of the three layers ectoderm, mesoderm and endoderm – induced by several proteins, the neural plate develops during embryonic week 3 as part of the ectoderm. Because of that, the ectoderm is divided into *surface* ectoderm and *neuro*ectoderm. The central parts of this neural plate fold and form the neural tube, later building the brain (including parts of the eyes) and the spinal cord. Some cells of the lateral borders of the neural plate differentiate into the so-called neural crest cells, which migrate into the underlying mesoderm and may therefore also be called "mesectoderm".

After embryonic week 3, organogenesis starts. From both walls of the diencephalon, which is the posterior part of the prosencephalon (forebrain), both optic vesicles evaginate. The optic vesicles, which consist of neuroectoderm, invaginate to double-layered optic cups and are connected to the brain by the optic stalk. The inner layer gives rise to the neural layers of the retina, the outer layer gives rise to the pigmented epithelium of the retina. Proteins induce the formation of the lens from the surface ectoderm. Each optic cup shows a groove, the choroidal fissure, on its undersurface. This groove is filled with mesodermal cells, which differentiate into the hyaloid artery and vein, later becoming the central retinal artery and vein. Between weeks 5 and 7, this groove closes to form the optic nerve with the axons of the retinal ganglion cells.

4.1 Embryology of the Parts of the Chamber Angle

Iris: The pigmented epithelium and its dorsal basal membrane develop from the inner layer of the optic cup (neuroectoderm). The sphincter (month 4) and dilator (month 6) pupillae muscles develop from the outer layer of the optic cup. The stroma with vessels, nerves, collagen fibers and chromatophores develop from the neural crest cells (mesectoderm).

Cornea: The epithelium develops from the surface ectoderm. Bowman layer and stroma, and the endothelium develop from the neural crest cells.

Sclera: The sclera develops from the neural crest cells (week 7). It is continuous with the corneal stroma anteriorly and with the dura posteriorly.

Anterior chamber: A group of neural crest cells is separated into two layers by vacuolization during month 3 by the growth of the rim of the optic cup centrally. The anterior cells form the corneal stroma and endothelium, and the posterior cells form the iridopupillary membrane, which is normally resorbed before birth. Sometimes remnants are visible as persistent pupillary membrane filaments (Fig. 4.1).

Trabecular meshwork, Schlemm's canal: Neural crest cells of the posterior area of the cornea form the trabecular meshwork during weeks 5–7. The cells evolute to typical trabecular cells of the uveal and corneoscleral trabeculum. Only the

C. Faschinger, A. Hommer, *Gonioscopy*,
DOI 10.1007/978-3-642-28610-0_4, © Springer-Verlag Berlin Heidelberg 2012

cribriform layer remains as unchanged neural crest cells for life. Schlemm's canal appears during month 4. This appearance depends on the growth of vessels from outside the sclera to the trabeculum. The month 5 is considered to be the start of the aqueous humor dynamics. Important for regular development of the opening of the chamber angle and its cleavage is a posterior movement, away from the cornea, starting during month 7.

Ciliary body: The epithelium of the ciliary body and the ciliary processes is double-layered (inner nonpigmented and outer pigmented) and develops from both layers of the optic cup (neuroectoderm). The processes grow and reach the equator of the lens forming fine filaments, the zonules. The processes produce the aqueous humor from month 4 onwards. The stroma and the ciliary muscle develop from the neural crest cells during month 7.

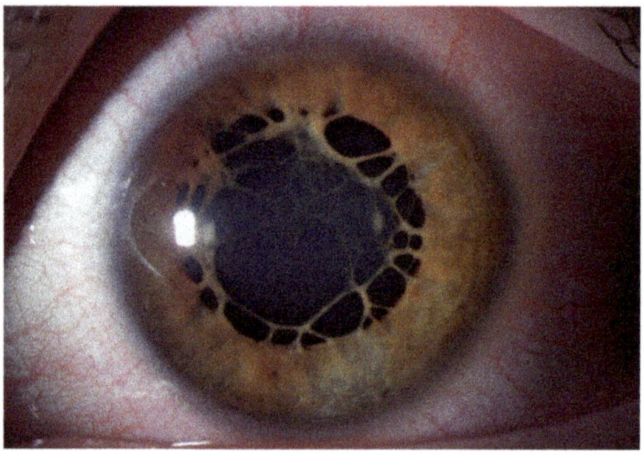

Fig. 4.1 Remnants of a formerly completely closed iridopupillary membrane, which is normally resorbed before birth, resembling a spider's web

Lens: The lens develops from the surface ectoderm. The hyaloid artery and annular vessels form the tunica vasculosa lentis for nutrition. During month 8 this vascular meshwork disappears.

The development of the different structures of the anterior segment of the eye is shown in Table 4.1.

The regular development of the outflow pathways depends on the maturation and formation of a porous trabecular meshwork, the ingrowth of Schlemm's canal and the posterior movement of the iris root. It is well known that the development of the chamber angle continues after birth.

If there is no regular development, different genotypic and phenotypic anomalies or syndromes will occur. They are called anterior chamber cleavage syndromes, neural crest dysgeneses or anterior segment dysgeneses, a heterogeneous family of diseases (formerly called "dysgenesis mesodermalis"). If the irregular development is combined with developmental disorders of other organs, then these anomalies are called syndromes.

In newborns and infants you need general anesthesia for appropriate examinations of the globe and the ocular structures. Take your time to do it as exactly as possible. Look closely and document well!

The chamber angle of a healthy eye of an infant differs from that of a healthy eye of an adult:

Table 4.1 Development of the different structures of the anterior segment of the eye

Ectoderm	Surface ectoderm		Lens
			Corneal epithelium
	Neuroectoderm	Neural plate → tube	Brain → optic vesicles
			Iris epithelium
			Iris muscles
			Ciliary body epithelium
		Neural crest cells ("mesectoderm")	Iris stroma
			Corneal stroma, endothelium, Schwalbe's ring
			Sclera, scleral spur
			Trabecular meshwork, Schlemm's canal
			Ciliary body stroma, ciliary muscle
Mesoderm			Vessels

- Almost no or very little pigment of the trabecular meshwork. The surface glistens like cellophane.
- Schwalbe's ring and the scleral spur are not as white as in adults.
- The recess is (much) smaller than in adults.
- The peripheral anterior stroma of the iris is thin, and the pigmented layer shines through.

4.2 Examples of Genetic Disorders of the Anterior Segment

4.2.1 Primary Congenital Glaucoma, Hydrophthalmus, Buphthalmus, Childhood Glaucoma (Birth to the 10th Year of Life)

The simplest developmental disorder is dysgenesis of the trabecular meshwork and Schlemm's canal (trabeculodysgenesis) that leads to hydrophthalmus or buphthalmus. The globe has a larger diameter than the age percentile values. The cornea has a diameter of more than 12 mm at birth and shows Haab's striae. There are breaks in Descemet's membrane running horizontally or parallel to the limbus (Fig. 4.2).

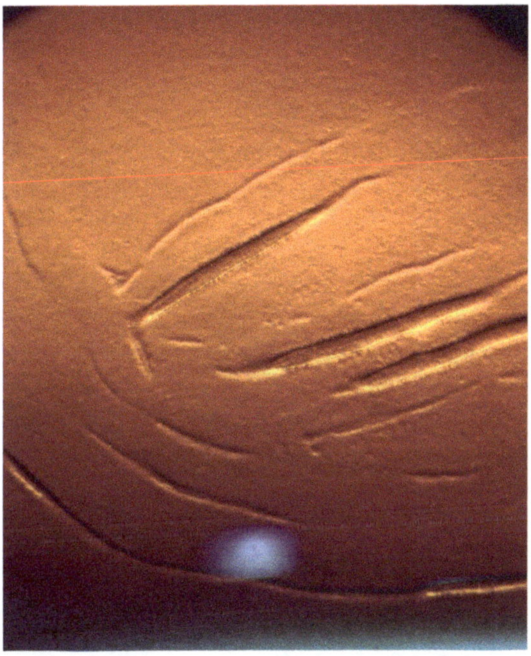

Fig. 4.2 Breaks in Descemet's membrane called Haab's striae in the cornea of an eye with buphthalmus (regredient light)

The chamber angle is open and it is not possible to differentiate the structures in detail. It is often combined with an anterior insertion of the iris with many iris processes. The neural crest cells have not developed properly to form the trabecular meshwork structures. Sometimes even Schlemm's canal is missing. The stroma of the peripheral iris is very hypoplastic and forms garlands, so you can easily detect the dark pigmented posterior layer of the iris (Fig. 4.3). An impermeable membrane, formerly called Barkan's membrane, coating the chamber angle, cannot be found histologically.

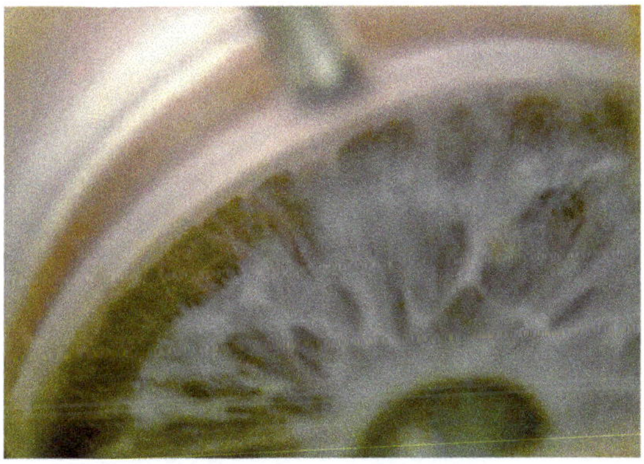

Fig. 4.3 Chamber angle in an eye with primary congenital glaucoma showing a scalloped appearance, prominent vessels on the iris, and a fine white membrane over the iris (special wide angle goniolens for goniotomy; courtesy P. Khaw)

The onset of the disease differs. It occurs bilaterally in 70%. In 80% it is diagnosed within the first year of life. If onset is later (after 3 or 4 years of age), the disease does not lead to a larger diameter of the globe because of the higher stiffness of the collagens of the sclera and cornea.

Besides sporadic cases, hereditary congenital glaucoma is associated with mutations in the genes CYP1B1 (coding for cytochrome P 450 1B1) and LTBP2 (latent transforming growth factor beta binding protein 2).

An eye with a megalocornea has a diameter larger than usual, but the anterior segment (cornea, iris and iris insertion, chamber angle) and all other parameters (IOP, optic disc, length of the globe) are within the normal ranges.

4.2.2 More Complex Dysgeneses: Secondary Childhood Glaucomas

Axenfeld described a prominent Schwalbe's ring and called it *embryotoxon corneae posterius*. It does not increase the risk for glaucoma. This white line often has connections to the anterior layer of the iris composed of fine thin fibers (Figs. 4.4, 4.5, and 4.6).

Rieger described the *dysgenesis mesodermalis corneae et iridis* with atrophy of the iris and an ectopic pupil due to adhesions or bridging tissue bands between the iris and (the prominent) Schwalbe's ring (Fig. 4.7).

Axenfeld-Rieger syndrome (autosomal dominant) shows developmental disorders of the anterior segment of the eye. Systemic disorders are dental and maxillary hypoplasia and failure of involution of the periumbilical skin. There are three types according to the pathological gene map locus: type 1 (RIEG1) with the locus on chromosome 4q25–q26, type 2 (RIEG2) with the locus on chromosome 13q14, and type 3 (RIEG3) with the locus on chromosome 6p25 (with cardiac defects).

Peters described congenital defects of Descemet's membrane presenting as a central corneal leucoma with circular synechiae around the center

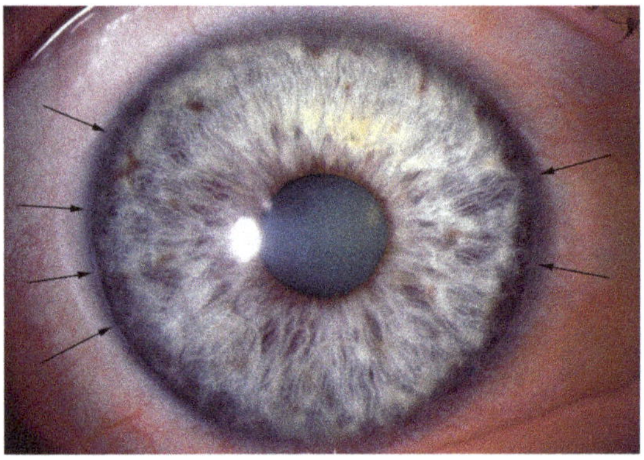

Fig. 4.4 Embryotoxon posterius is seen as a thin *white line* in the nasal and temporal parts of the peripheral cornea (*arrows*) and represents a prominent Schwalbe's ring. It is of no pathological concern in relation to glaucoma

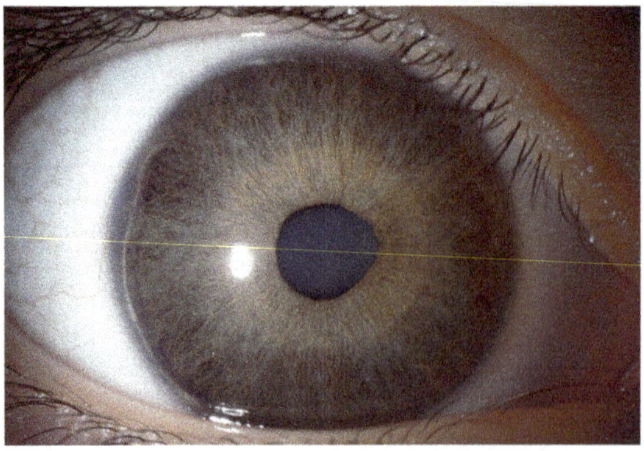

Fig. 4.5 Slitlamp photograph of a prominent Schwalbe's ring temporally

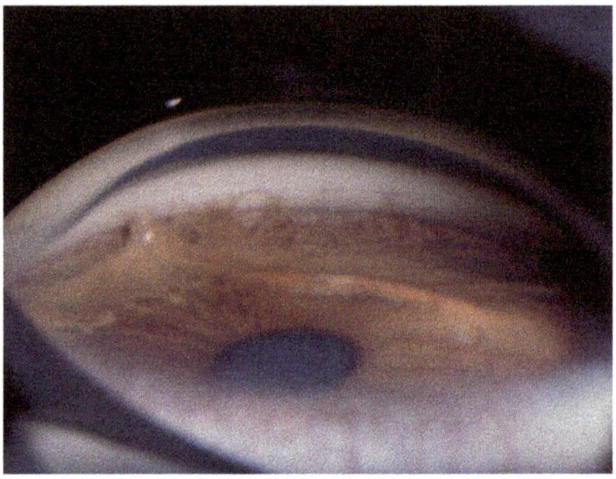

Fig. 4.6 Gonioscopic findings of the eye in Fig. 4.5 showing tissue bridges from the iris to the prominent Schwalbe's ring (embryotoxon posterius)

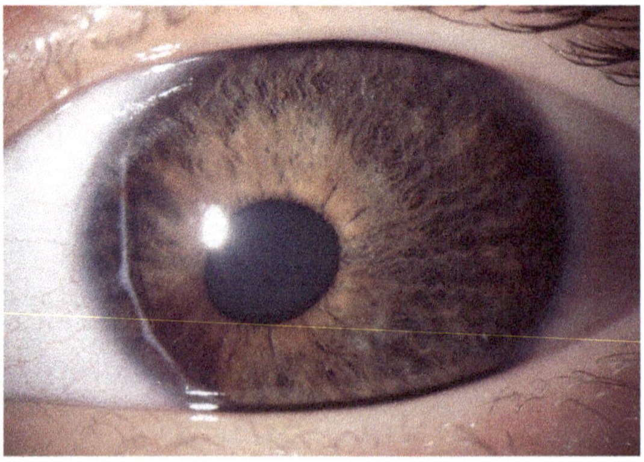

Fig. 4.7 Rieger anomaly with *white line* in the nasal periphery of the cornea with bridging tissue bands decentering the pupil (korectopia)

of the cornea, and a missing deep corneal stroma, Descemet's membrane and endothelium centrally. Surgical treatment is generally unsuccessful and these eyes have a very poor prognosis (Figs. 4.8 and 4.9).

In aniridia the amount of missing iris tissue is variable. Even if most of the iris is absent, a small amount of iris tissue is always present, which is mostly torn forward closing the trabecular meshwork of the chamber angle leading to secondary angle closure glaucoma (Fig. 4.10). The gene map locus is on chromosome 11p13. In sporadic aniridia with large deletions of the chromosome the probability of developing a Wilms tumor is high.

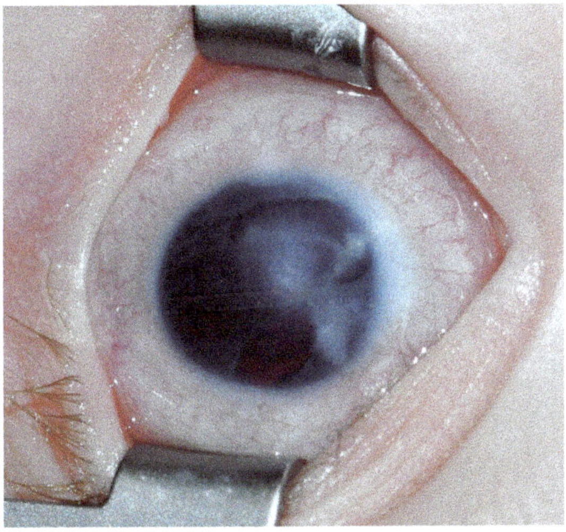

Fig. 4.8 Right eye of a baby with Peters anomaly showing dense central leucomas of the cornea due to misdevelopment of the inner structures with anterior synechiae and iris holes

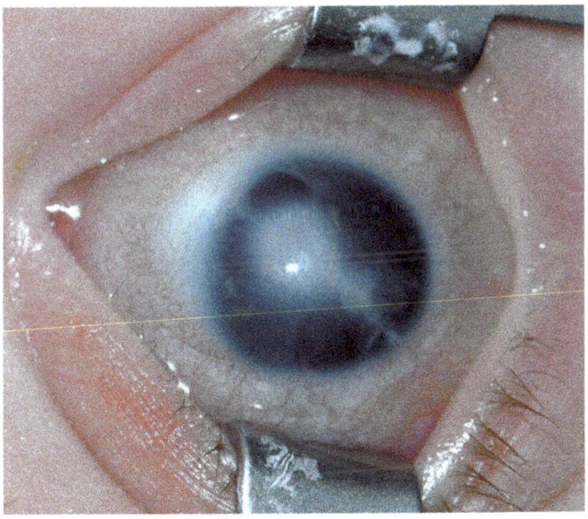

Fig. 4.9 Left eye of the baby in Fig. 4.8 with Peters anomaly showing dense central leucomas of the cornea due to misdevelopment of the inner structures with anterior synechiae and iris holes

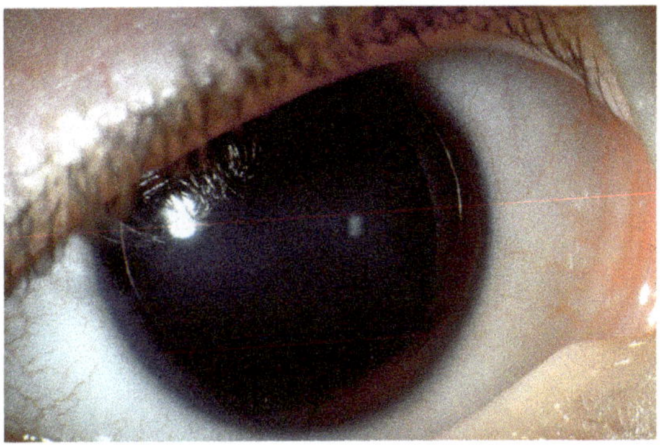

Fig. 4.10 Aniridia with visible margins of the lens as golden reflex nasally and temporally. Usually there are small remnants of iris tissue in the chamber angle

All these dysgenetic disorders have a risk of blindness of about 50% due to glaucoma, despite many attempts to regulate the IOP.

Several other diseases of the eye may lead to a pediatric glaucoma: aphakia (especially when operated on before week 8 after birth), persistent primary hyperplastic vitreous, retinopathy of prematurity, ectopia of the lens, microspherophakia, microphthalmus, phacomatoses, inflammations, tumors, etc.

Bibliography

Axenfeld T (1920) Embryotoxon corneae posterius. Berichte der Deutschen Ophthalmologischen Gesellschaft 42: 301–302

Azar NF, Davis EA (1999) Embryology of the eye. In: Yanoff M, Duker JS (eds) Ophthalmology. Mosby, London

Lagreze W (2011) Glaukom im Säuglings- und Kindesalter. Diagnostik und Therapie. Z prakt Augenheilkd 32: 364–368

Online Mendelian Inheritance in Man (OMIM). http://www.ncbi.nlm.nih.gov/omim

Peters A (1906) Über angeborene Defektbildung der Descemetschen Membran. Klin Monatsbl Augenheilkd 44(27–40):105–119

Reese AB, Ellsworth RM (1966) The anterior cleavage syndrome. Arch Ophthalmol 75:307–318

Reis LM, Semina EV (2011) Genetics of anterior segment dysgenesis disorders. Curr Opin Ophthalmol 22:314–324

Rieger H (1935) Beiträge zur Kenntnis seltener Missbildungen der Iris: über Hypoplasie des Irisvorderblattes mit Verlagerung und Entrundung der Pupille. Graefes Arch Clin Exp Ophthalmol 133:602–635

Tamm ER (2011) Entwicklung des Kammerwinkels und kongenitales Glaukom. Ophthalmologe 108: 610–617

Wang D, Wang M, Console JW, He M, Seider MI, Lin SC (2009) Distinctive findings in a patient with Axenfeld-Rieger syndrome using high-resolution AS-OCT. Ophthalmic Surg Lasers Imaging 40:589–592

5 Grading Systems and Documentation

5.1 Gonioscopic Grading Systems

Grading systems are necessary to define the diagnosis of open-angle or angle-closure glaucoma. They help to estimate the risk of development of an angle-closure or angle-closure attack. To describe the width of the chamber angle, i.e., the distance between the anterior surface of the peripheral roll of the iris and the posterior trabecular meshwork, several grading systems have been established. The grading in an eye might change over time and it is therefore important in follow-up.

The major problem is that the chamber angle is not an angle per se but is a recess, since there is a distance between the iris root and the junction between the ciliary band and the posterior trabecular meshwork.

Gradle and Sugar (1940) were the first to measure the depth of the anterior chamber and they calculated the apparent "angle-wall depth" by drawing an imaginary line from Schwalbe's ring perpendicular to the iris. Eyes with "uncompensated" glaucoma had smaller values than normal eyes or eyes with "compensated" glaucoma or glaucoma capsulare. They called their method goniometry, but they did not grade the eyes.

Always ask yourself: is the angle open or closed? If it is closed, is it by appositions or synechiae? If it is open, is it occludable?

5.1.1 Scheie (1957)

This system is based on the visibility of the anatomical structures of the angle and includes five categories (Table 5.1). A wide open angle was graded as Wide, a slightly narrowed as grade I, the apex (i.e. ciliary body) not visible as II, the posterior half of the trabeculum not visible as III, and none of the angle visible as IV.

5.1.2 Shaffer (1960)

This system is based on angularity. Shaffer wanted to avoid confusion because at that time two methods of classifying angles by numbers were used, but in one system (Scheie) "grade I" was an open angle, and in the second system Sugar (1957) "grade 1" was an almost closed angle. He suggested that an anatomical classification without numbers be used (Table 5.2). Wide open angles have an opening in the range 45–20°, and narrow angles in the range 20–0°. A shallow anterior chamber with a narrow angle less than 20° open

Table 5.1 Grading system of Scheie

Grade	Visibility of structures	Interpretation
Wide	Wide	Wide open, all structures visible
I	Slightly narrowed	Ciliary body visible, but recess obscured by the last roll of the iris
II	Apex not visible	Ciliary body not visible
III	Posterior half of trabeculum not visible	Ciliary body, scleral spur and posterior half of the trabeculum not visible
IV	None of the angle visible	Ciliary body, scleral spur, trabeculum not visible

C. Faschinger, A. Hommer, *Gonioscopy*,
DOI 10.1007/978-3-642-28610-0_5, © Springer-Verlag Berlin Heidelberg 2012

Table 5.2 Grading system of Shaffer (1960)

Classification	Clinical interpretation
1. Wide open angle	Closure improbable or impossible
2. Narrow angle, moderate	Closure possible
3. Narrow angle, extreme	Closure probable, eventually
4. Narrow angle, closed (complete or partial)	Angle closure present

Table 5.3 Anatomical grading system of Shaffer (1962)

Angular grade	Width	Grade	Clinical interpretation
Wide open angle	45–35°	4	Angle closure impossible
	35–20°	3	Angle closure impossible
Narrow angle	20°	2	Angle closure possible
Narrow angle, extreme	10° or less	1	Angle closure probable, eventually
Narrow angle, slit	Critically narrowed angle, quit possibly against trabecular meshwork beyond Schwalbe's line		
Narrow angle, partial or complete closure	0°	0	Angle closed in part or all of circumference

was considered as representing the risk of angle closure and/or pupillary block.

5.1.3 Shaffer (1962)

Two years later Shaffer presented a numerical grading system with grades from 0 to 4 (Table 5.3). These numbers should not be mixed up with those of Scheie! In the Scheie system, grade 1 is an open angle, and in the Shaffer system, grade 1 is a very narrow angle recess.

5.1.4 Spaeth

To emphasize the complexity of the recess and the angle configurations, Spaeth proposed a system integrating the iris insertion, angularity, configuration and the pigmentation of the posterior trabecular meshwork.

- Iris insertion: designated *A* (anterior to the trabecular meshwork), *B* (between Schwalbe's ring and scleral spur or behind Schwalbe's ring), *C* (at the scleral spur), *D* (deep), or *E* (extremely deep) (see Chap. 3, Fig. 3.15).
- Iris angularity: (10–40°): estimation in degrees might be more difficult than relying on visible or invisible structures. It is difficult to place a tangent on the iris because the curvature is rarely totally flat, and it might be convex or concave. Spaeth proposed that the first line be drawn as a tangent to the inner surface of the trabecular meshwork and the second line as a tangent to the anterior iris surface approximately one-third of the distance from the most peripheral portion of the iris (Fig. 5.1)
- Iris configuration: designated *S* (steep), or *b* (bowing anteriorly), *p* plateau configuration, *R* regular, or *f* flat without bowing, *c* concave posteriorly with bowing (see Chap. 3, Fig. 3.16).
- Pigmentation (ptm) of the trabecular meshwork: graded 0–4 (see Sect. 5.1.1 Scheie)

  Examples:

  D40f 1ptm: angle with a deep iris insertion, 40° angulation, a flat iris and pigmentation grade 1. This is a normal angle.

  A40f 1ptm: angle with an anterior iris insertion, 40° angulation and a flat iris. This is the case in synechiae or neovascular glaucoma.

  D40c 4ptm: angle with a deep iris insertion, 40° angulation, a concave posteriorly bowing and highly pigmented posterior trabecular meshwork. This might be the case in high myopia (less pigment) or in pigment dispersion syndrome.

  (B)D30p 0ptm: angle with iris insertion between Schwalbe's line and scleral spur (value in in parentheses means that it was determined first without indentation). After indentation gonioscopy, the angle was classified as deep insertion of the iris, 30° angulation, plateau configuration, and no

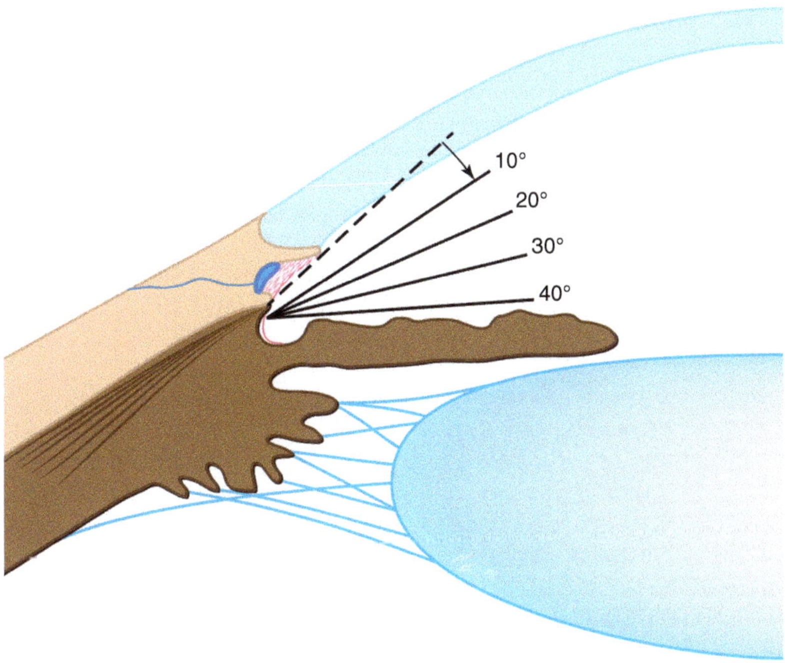

Fig. 5.1 The first (reference) line (*dashed line*) is a tangent to the inner surface of the trabecular meshwork, and the second line is a tangent to the anterior iris surface approximately one-third of the distance from the most peripheral portion of the iris

Table 5.4 Grading system of Becker

	0	1	2	3
0	Angle closed	Small trabecular zone, iris insertion not visible	Average width of trabecular zone, iris insertion not visible	Broad trabecular zone, iris insertion not visible
A		Small trabecular zone, iris insertion anteriorly	Average width of trabecular zone, iris insertion anteriorly	Broad trabecular zone, iris insertion anteriorly
B		Small trabecular zone, iris insertion in the middle	Average width of trabecular zone, iris insertion in the middle	Broad trabecular zone, iris insertion in the middle
C		Small trabecular zone, iris insertion posteriorly	Average width of trabecular zone, iris insertion posteriorly	Broad trabecular zone, iris insertion posteriorly

pigment. This is an angle in plateau iris configuration.

5.1.5 Becker

In this classification two points are of main interest: first the width of the trabecular zone between Schwalbe's ring and the scleral spur, and second the distance between the scleral spur and insertion of the iris (Table 5.4). The numbers indicate the width of the trabecular zone, and the letters insertion of the iris. A chamber angle classified as *1-A* means that the angle is open, a small zone of trabecular meshwork is visible and insertion of the iris is anterior. A classification of 3-C means that the angle is wide open with a broad trabecular zone and insertion of the iris is posterior.

5.1.6 Shaffer-Kanski

This is a practicable grading system based on the angularity width described by Shaffer and the visibility of the structures, and is relevant to the risk of an angle closure (Table 5.5).

Remember: The width of the chamber angle need not be the same throughout the 360° circumference. If it varies, document the width for each quadrant.

Table 5.5 Grading system of Shaffer-Kanski

Grade	Angle (°)	Visibility of structures	Risk of angle closure
0	0	No structures visible	Closed angle
1	About 10	Schwalbe's line, possibly anterior, nonfunctional trabecular meshwork visible	Closure possible
2	20	Schwalbe's line and trabecular meshwork visible	Narrow, closure unlikely
3	20–35	Schwalbe's line, trabecular meshwork and scleral spur visible	Closure impossible
4	35–45	All structures visible from Schwalbe's line to ciliary band	Closure impossible

Table 5.6 Grading system of Van Herick

Grade	Cornea: peripheral anterior chamber ratio	Risk of angle closure	Angle (°)
4[a]	1:1 or higher	Very unlikely or impossible	35–40
3	1:½	Unlikely or improbable	20–35
2	1:¼	Possible	20
1[b]	1:<¼	Likely or probable	10
0	No anterior chamber slit visible	Closed	0

[a]Illustrated in Fig. 5.2
[b]Illustrated in Fig. 5.3

5.2 Non-gonioscopic Grading Systems

5.2.1 Peripheral Anterior Chamber (Van Herick Method)

This non-gonioscopic estimation of the depth of the *peripheral* anterior chamber also provides information on the width of the chamber angle. It is easily done with the slit lamp and it is helpful before dilating a pupil for diagnostic and therapeutic reasons (for example, in patients who need laser treatment for diabetic retinopathy or peripheral retinal degeneration).

Use a slim beam coming from the periphery (60° angularity of the slit lamp) and put it on the periphery of the cornea, not far from the limbus. Calculate the ratio between the thickness of the slit of the cornea (reference value 1) and the depth of the anterior chamber (second value 2). The system is shown in Table 5.6, and example slit lamp images are shown in Figs. 5.2 and 5.3.

This evaluation does not replace gonioscopy, because no structures are identified, but it is highly informative, and is quickly done without an additional instrument (lens) or any discomfort for the patient.

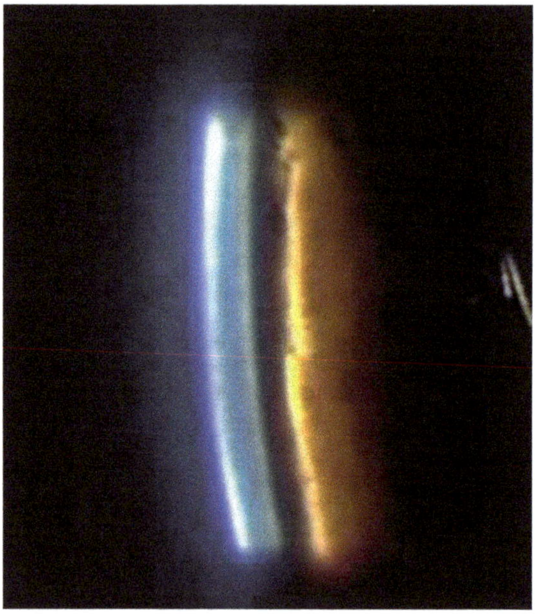

Fig. 5.2 Normal depth of the peripheral anterior chamber (grade 4). The cornea and peripheral chamber are of equal thickness (ratio 1:1)

5.2.2 Central Anterior Chamber (Ghorbani-Smith Method)

This method gives the depth of the *central* anterior chamber.

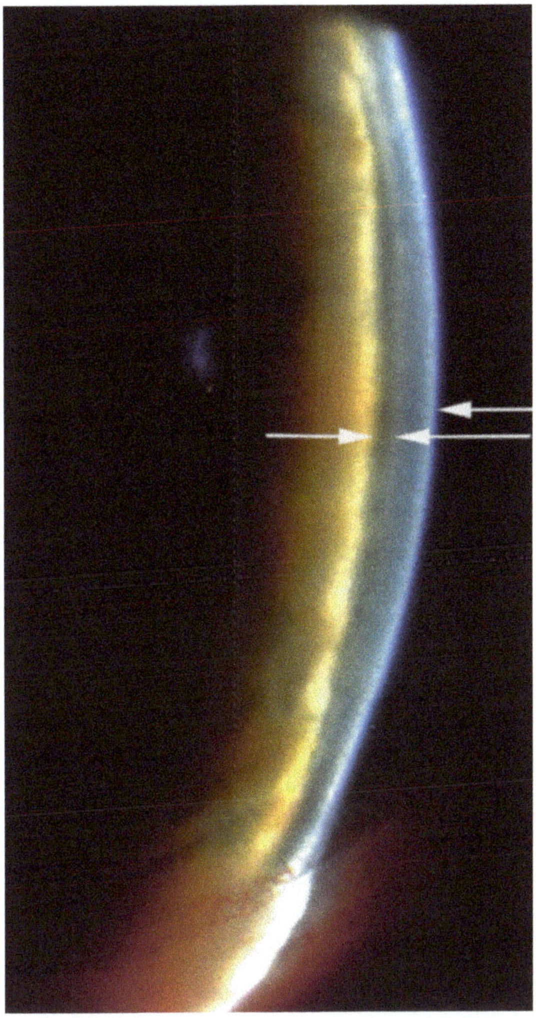

Fig. 5.3 Very shallow peripheral anterior chamber. The *two left-pointing arrows* indicate the thickness of the cornea, the *right-pointing arrow* the iris, *between the two long arrows* indicates the depth of the peripheral anterior chamber. The ratio between the depth and the thickness of the cornea is less than one quarter (Van Herick 1). These pupils should not be dilated without checking the IOP after a few hours

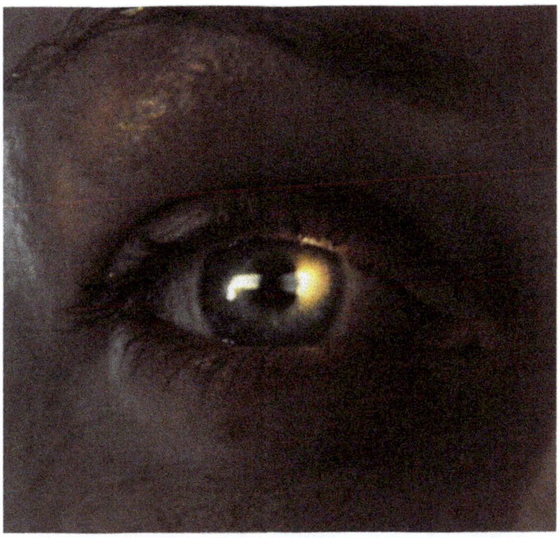

Fig. 5.4 Horizontal slit of the slitlamp focused at the cornea and unfocused on the surface of the iris or lens. The slitlamp is 60° off-center to the left in a left eye

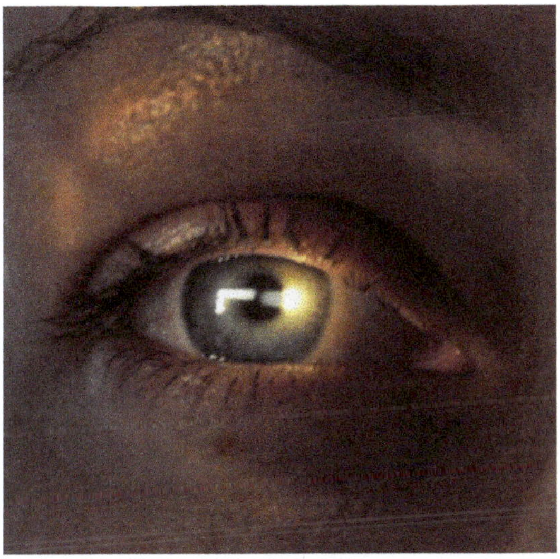

Fig. 5.5 By increasing the length of the slit the two slits will almost meet

Use the slit lamp and at first adjust the slit in a horizontal position. Fix the arm of the slit lamp temporally at 60°. The microscope is pointed straight ahead and the patient is asked to look straight ahead. Shorten the slit to 1–2 mm and move the slit lamp until it is focused at the cornea. You will find a second slit on the surface of the iris and/or the lens (depending on the width of the pupil), that is slightly unfocused (Fig. 5.4). Increase the length of the slit until the two slits meet (Figs. 5.5 and 5.6). Read the length at the scale of the slit lamp (Fig. 5.7) and multiply this value by 1.4 (for values between 1 and 2.5 mm) or add 10% of the value and 0.5 mm. This will give you the central anterior chamber depth (corneal endothelium to the anterior surface of the lens) in millimeters. An eye with a central chamber depth of 2 mm or less is at risk of developing

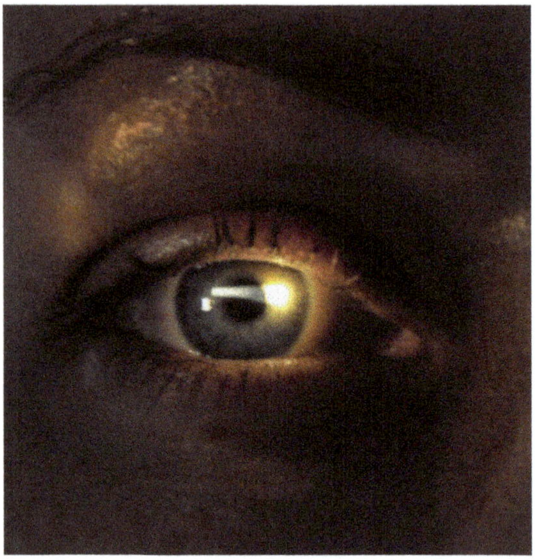

Fig. 5.6 The two slits meet – finished

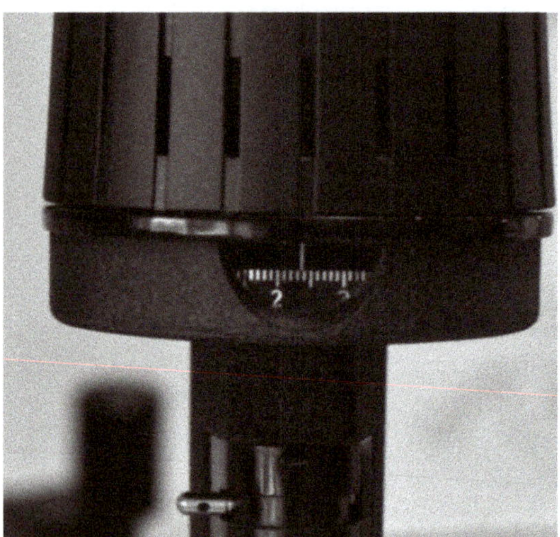

Fig. 5.7 Read the value from the scale

angle closure. If you measure the right eye you must only use the right ocular and vice versa for the left eye.

5.2.3 Additional Procedures in Gonioscopy

The chamber angle can also be analyzed using several additional procedures including anterior segment optical coherence tomography (AS-OCT), ultrasound biomicroscopy (UBM) and Pentacam-Scheimpflug imaging. These procedures and their sophisticated software provide useful parameters including the width of the chamber angle and anterior chamber volume and nicely show the relative positions of the iris, lens and cornea (see Chap. 8).

5.3 Documentation of the Structures of the Chamber Angle

Your interpretations and drawings of the chamber angle need to be understandable by other ophthalmologists.

The most important part of the chamber angle is the functional, posterior trabecular meshwork. If it is partially or totally covered by iris tissue, then angle closure is definitely present. So you have to document whether the trabecular meshwork is seen or not seen, adding the number of degrees where it is visible.

Increase the validity by adding the depth of the central anterior chamber (less or more than 2 mm) and the width of the pupil during examination. Add the peripheral configuration of the iris (*Q* queer or *c* concave, *R* regular or *f* flat, *S* steep or convex or *b* bowing forward) and the peripheral insertion of the iris (*A*, *B*, *C*, *D*, *E*). For the angle width use the grading system you are used to. If you perform dynamic or indentation gonioscopy, document the results, e.g. *IG open* in indentation gonioscopy the iridocorneal appositions are opened, or *IG closed* in indentation gonioscopy the angle remains closed (this is synechial closure).

You may also use the sophisticated documentation suggested by Spaeth.

Besides a written description, you can also include a drawn diagram of the chamber angle.

We suggest that you draw a circle and divide it in four sectors of 90°: superior, nasal, inferior, temporal. Inside each sector you designate the most posterior structure of the chamber angle that is visible (*SS* for scleral spur visible but anterior ciliary band not visible; *TM* for trabecular meshwork visible but scleral spur not visible, etc.). You can add the grade of the pigmentation (Scheie 0–4). Details about the iris (insertion, angularity, configuration) are not included.

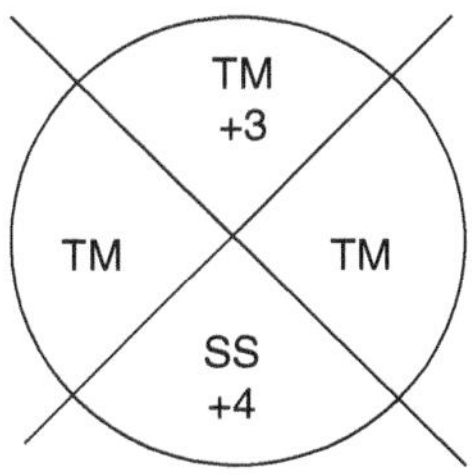

Or you can use numbers, but be sure not to mix up the different grading systems. Inside each sector you can insert the grade of the angle opening (e.g., Shaffer) and outside each sector you can add specific findings, such as PAS, new vessels, etc.

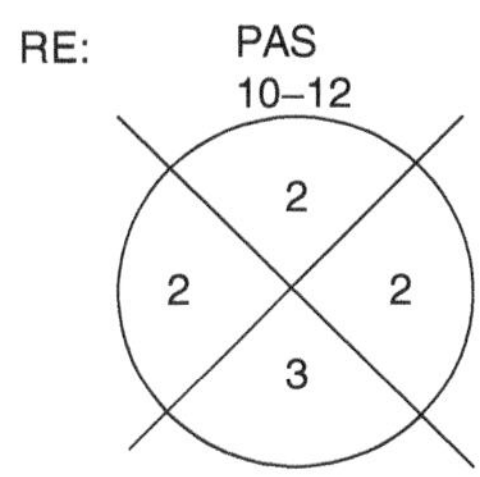

Bibliography

Alward WL, Longmuir RA (2008) Color atlas of gonioscopy, 2nd edn. American Academy of Ophthalmology, San Francisco

Becker SC, Grüning HD (1976) Gonioskopie. Lehrbuch und Atlas mit stereoskopischen Bildern. Schattauer, Stuttgart

Douthwaite WA, Spence D (1986) Slit-lamp measurement of the anterior chamber depth. Br J Ophthalmol 70: 205–208

Gorban AI (1968) Optical-geometric method of determining the depth of the anterior chamber by means of slit lamp (ShChL-56). Vestn Oftalmol 81:77–80

Gradle HS, Sugar HS (1940) Concerning the chamber angle. III. A clinical method of goniometry. Am J Ophthalmol 23:1135–1139

Hoskins HD, Kass MA (1989) Gonioscopy. In: Hoskins HD, Kass MA (eds) Becker-Shaffer's diagnosis and therapy of the glaucomas. CV Mosby, St. Louis

Kanski J, Spitznas M (1987) Glaukom. In: Kanski J, Spitznas M (eds) Lehrbuch der klinischen Ophthalmologie. Thieme, Stuttgart

Salmon JF (2009) Gonioscopy. In: Shaarawy TM, Sherwood MB, Hitchings RA, Crowston G (eds) Glaucoma, vol I. Saunders Elsevier, Philadelphia

Scheie HG (1957) Width and pigmentation of the angle of the anterior chamber. A system of grading by gonioscopy. Arch Ophthalmol 58:510–514

Shaffer RN (1960) Gonioscopy, ophthalmoscopy and perimetry. Trans Am Acad Ophthalmol Otolaryngol 64:112–127

Shaffer RN (1962) Gonioscopic anatomy of the angle of the anterior chamber of the eye. In: Shaffer RN (ed) Stereoscopic manual of gonioscopy. Mosby, St Louis, pp 29–39

Smith RJ (1979) A new method of estimating the depth of the anterior chamber. Br J Ophthalmol 63:215–220

Spaeth GL (1971) The normal development of the human anterior chamber angle: a new system of descriptive grading. Trans Ophthalmol Soc U K 91:709–739

Sugar HS (1957) The glaucomas. 1st ed. Hoeber-Harper, New York

Van Herick W, Shaffer RN, Schwartz A (1968) Estimation of width of angle of anterior chamber. Am J Ophthalmol 68:626–632

6 Open Angle and Glaucoma

6.1 The Chamber Angle in Primary Open-Angle Glaucoma or Ocular Hypertension with Open Angle

Etiology: Increased resistance to outflow in the cribriform or juxtacanalicular trabecular meshwork, building the inner wall of Schlemm's canal (trabecular dysfunction), and apoptosis of the retinal ganglion cells as well as degeneration of the optic nerve axons with alterations of connective tissues at the optic disc.

Chamber angle, iris and lens: Because of the invisibility of Schlemm's canal and the cribriform trabeculum, the chamber angle does not show any changes compared to an ordinary, regular angle. It is open and all structures are visible. It is the same in juvenile glaucoma, ocular hypertension, preperimetric glaucoma, high-tension or normal-tension glaucoma. The diagnostic value of gonioscopy in POAG is the finding of an open angle. It is a diagnosis by exclusion. This is indeed very important for differential diagnosis in relation to all other forms of glaucoma.

Note: On aging, the angle might become narrower and occludable due to an increase in the volume of the lens. If this happens, parts of the angle become invisible, for example the anterior ciliary band, the scleral spur, the trabecular meshwork and even Schwalbe's ring.

Perform dynamic indentation gonioscopy to distinguish these changes from an angle closure due to appositions or synechiae. In a case of a thick lens the iris will move only slightly and evenly backwards. The therapy of choice is phacoemulsification. No antiglaucomatous therapy, no filtration surgery!

Remember: Primary open-angle glaucoma (OAG) is a diagnosis of exclusion. There are plenty of diagnoses that have to be excluded.

6.2 The Chamber Angle in Secondary Open-Angle Glaucoma

Secondary OAGs are caused by ocular or extraocular diseases or are iatrogenic.

6.2.1 Open-Angle Glaucoma Caused by Ocular Diseases

6.2.1.1 Pseudoexfoliation Syndrome (PXS) and Glaucoma (PXG)

Etiology: Production and deposition of extracellular white fibrillar material by different cells (lens epithelial cells, ciliary epithelial cells, cells of the iris, corneal endothelial cells, cells of the trabecular meshwork) in the anterior segment of the eye.

Pathomechanism: Fibrillogranular proteinaceous material is produced in the eye, released into the aqueous humor and in combination with released pigment reduces the outflow in the trabecular meshwork by accumulation.

Chamber angle, iris and lens: This material is rubbed off of the anterior surface of the lens within a zone of medium width and released into

C. Faschinger, A. Hommer, *Gonioscopy*,
DOI 10.1007/978-3-642-28610-0_6, © Springer-Verlag Berlin Heidelberg 2012

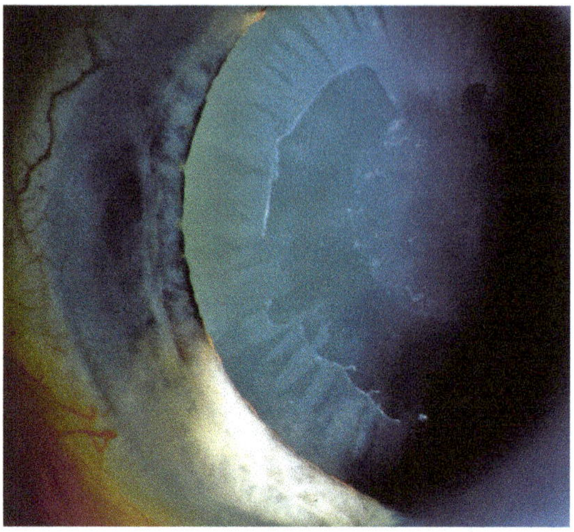

Fig. 6.1 Pseudoexfoliation material on the anterior surface of the lens, some of which has been rubbed off in the mid-periphery by the pupil

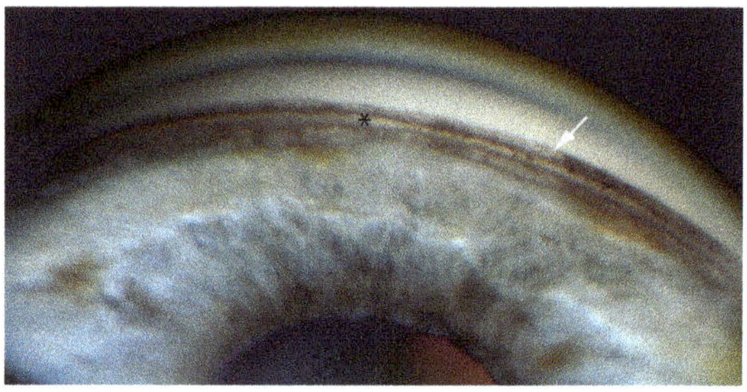

Fig. 6.2 Chamber angle of an eye with pseudoexfoliation (*arrow* white Schwalbe's ring). In the direction towards the cornea there is a very thin dark line (Sampaolesi's line). *Asterisk* indicates the bright white scleral spur. Between the scleral spur and Schwalbe's line is the pigmented trabecular meshwork (grade +3)

the aqueous humor (Fig. 6.1). It is also found on the zonular fibers, sometimes on the endothelium of the cornea, typically and easily recognized on the pigmented, brown pupillary margin of the iris and on the trabecular meshwork. The dark, pigmented epithelium of the iris is less tight, becomes loose and mixes with the white fibrillar material, producing a "salt and pepper" appearance in the trabecular meshwork. In addition Sampaolesi's line is often present in the inferior part or circumferentially (Figs. 6.2 and 6.3).

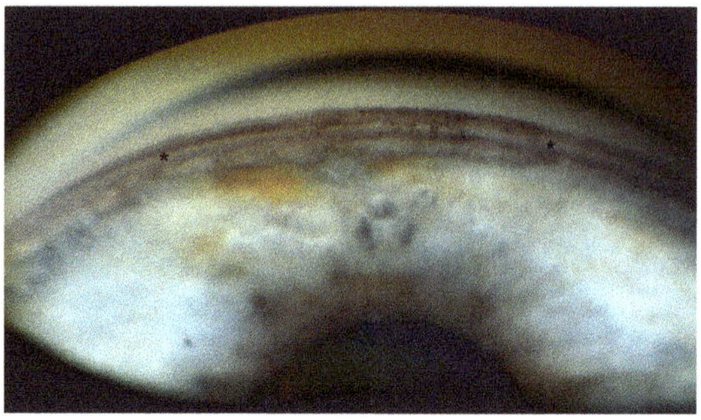

Fig. 6.3 Chamber angle of an eye with pseudoexfoliation (*asterisks* bright white scleral spur). Black pigment granules are present in the inferior part of the angle at 6 o'clock

Course: Due to weakening of the zonular fibers the lens can become subluxated (phacodonesis) resulting in a shallow or very deep anterior chamber and a narrow or very deep chamber angle. Narrow, occludable angles with pupillary block are more common. The IOP is higher and has a higher diurnal fluctuations than in primary OAG.

6.2.1.2 Pigment Dispersion Syndrome (PDS) and Pigmentary Glaucoma (PG)

Etiology: Pigmented epithelial cells (with melanin) rupture and pigment granules from the posterior surface of the iris are released and accumulate in the trabecular meshwork and in the endothelial trabecular cells.

Chamber angle, iris and lens: Posterior bowing of the peripheral parts of the iris result in a concave peripheral iris, a reverse pupillary block with higher pressure in the anterior chamber than in the posterior chamber. The peripheral pigmented layer of the iris will be rubbed off by the zonular fibers during movements of the pupil. This leads to radial transillumination defects or the so-called "church-window" phenomenon, seen as a crown-like red reflex of the fundus that resembles a rosetta window of a gothic church (Fig. 6.4). Pigmented cells are released into the aqueous humor and may be found on the anterior surface of the iris (Fig. 6.5). They are phagocytosed by the endothelial cells of the trabecular meshwork. This induces an intense or very intense brown pigmentation of the trabecular meshwork (Scheie grade +3 or +4), especially in the inferior part (Fig. 6.6). Additionally Sampaolesi's line is very often present. Vertical deposits of pigment on the corneal endothelium are called Krukenberg spindle (Fig. 6.7). Even the zonular fibers and the peripheral posterior surface of the lens (Scheie's stripe) are full of pigment cells (Fig. 6.8).

Course: The IOP shows high fluctuations. Over time – when accommodation is lost due to aging – most of the pigment has been released and the pigment dispersion or glaucoma has "burned out". Then the pigmentation of the trabecular meshwork becomes less in the inferior part and more prominent in the superior half ("pigment reversal").

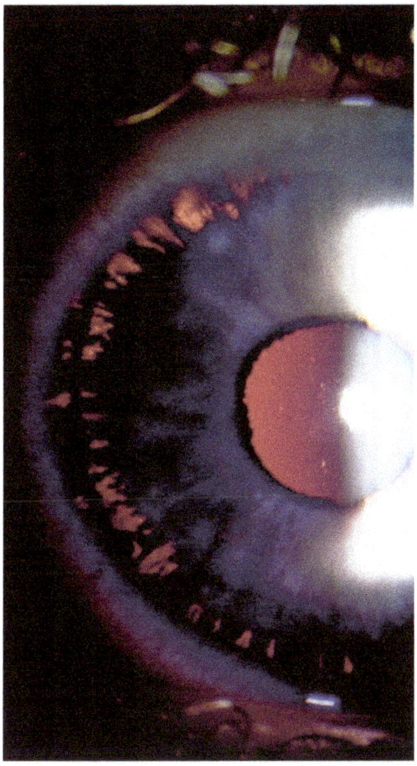

Fig. 6.4 Transillumination of the iris. Peripheral pigment is rubbed off by the movement of the pigmented layer of the iris on the zonular fibers

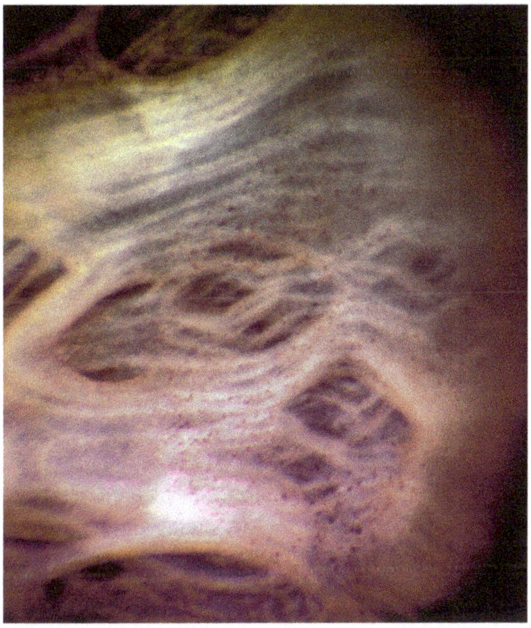

Fig. 6.5 Pigment on the anterior layer of the iris

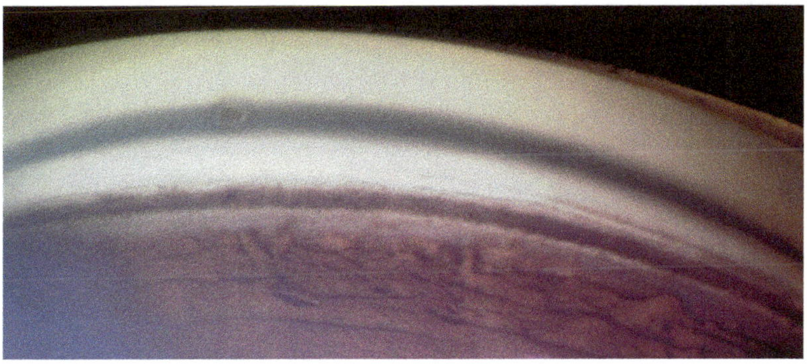

Fig. 6.6 Deep and wide open chamber angle of an eye with pigmentary glaucoma showing a highly pigmented trabecular meshwork between the scleral spur and Schwalbe's ring, and a broad ciliary band

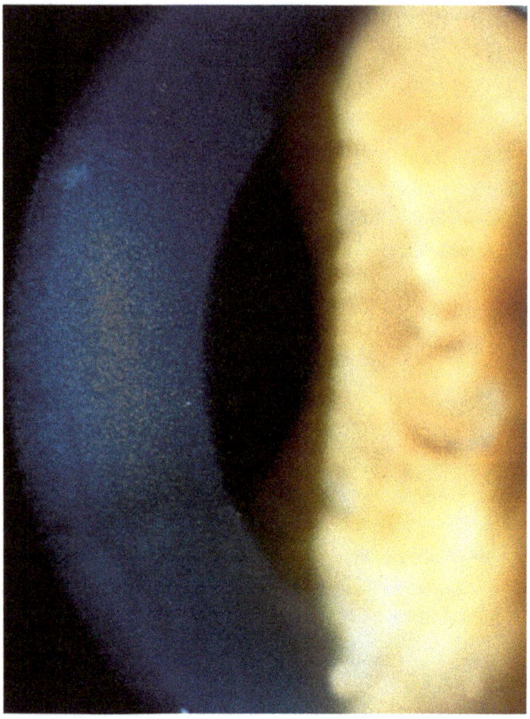

Fig. 6.7 Pigment granules on the endothelial side of the cornea in a spindle-like shape (Krikenberg)

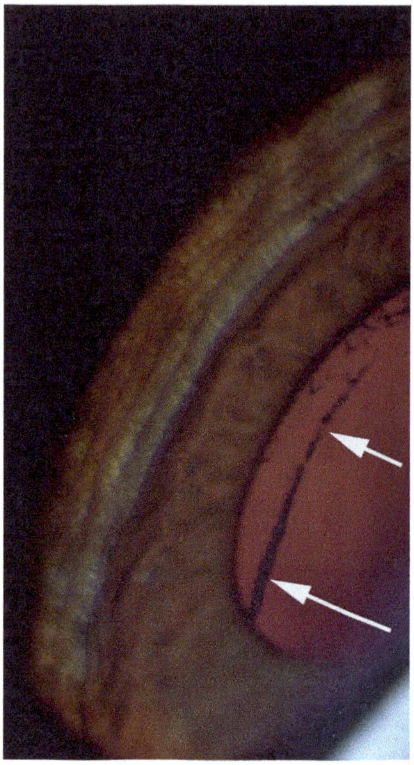

Fig. 6.8 Linear pigment deposits on the posterior surface of the lens, called Scheie's stripe (*arrows*). They are located peripherally to Wieger's ligament, the circular adhesion of the vitreous body on the lens

Note: In a very concave configuration of the peripheral iris a reverse pupillary block exists and a peripheral iridotomy may be indicated. The pigmented material will not pour into the anterior chamber as usually seen in angle closure. It appears to be reversed from the anterior to the posterior chamber due to pressure difference; it looks like the action of a vacuum cleaner. A second indication for an iridotomy may be an increase in the IOP 2–4 h after dilation of the pupil and an increase in pigment release to the anterior chamber. After iridotomy the formerly concave shape of the iris resolves. UBM and/or AS-OCT may be helpful in confirming the posterior bowing of the peripheral iris (Fig. 6.9).

6.2.1.3 Lens-Induced Secondary Open-Angle Glaucoma

Etiology/pathomechanisms: Lens matter or inflammatory cells induced by lens proteins. Conditions in which this occurs include: lens particle glaucoma (after penetrating or perforating trauma of the lens capsule); phacolytic glaucoma (mature or hypermature cataract releases lens proteins; Figs. 6.10 and 6.11); and phacoanaphylaxis (lens proteins released during uneventful cataract surgery of a first eye sensitizes the body leading to inflammation when the second eye is operated upon).

Chamber angle: Mainly the inferior part will show some lens material when the capsule is injured.

6.2.1.4 Red Blood Cells

Etiology/pathomechanisms: Fresh red blood cells (hyphema, Fig. 6.12) or old red blood cells (i.e. ghost cells 120 days after an intraocular hemorrhage) or a large quantity of red blood cells (sickle-cell disease) will obstruct the outflow of the trabecular meshwork.

Chamber angle: During resorption of a hyphema the blood in Schlemm's canal will be visible through the trabecular meshwork. Ghost

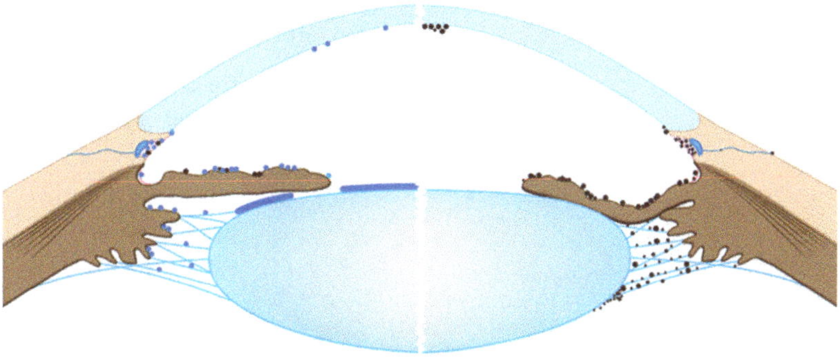

Fig. 6.9 Schematic drawing showing the differences in pseudoexfoliation (*left*, *blue* is pseudoexfoliative material) and pigment dispersion (*brown* is released pigment)

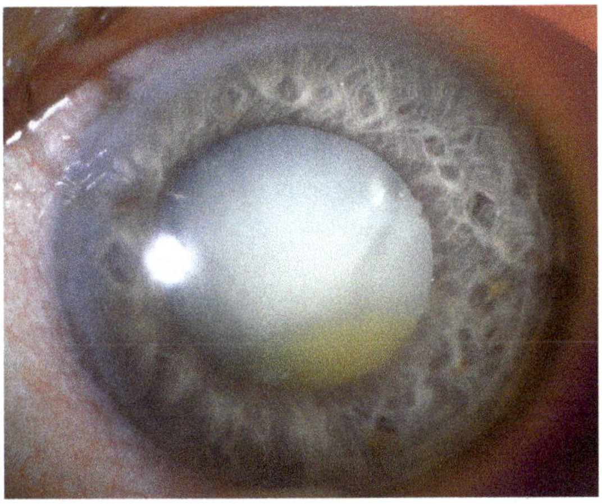

Fig. 6.10 Hypermature cataract with small brown nucleus, and a slightly hazy cornea in the inferior half due to higher IOP (phacolytic hypertension)

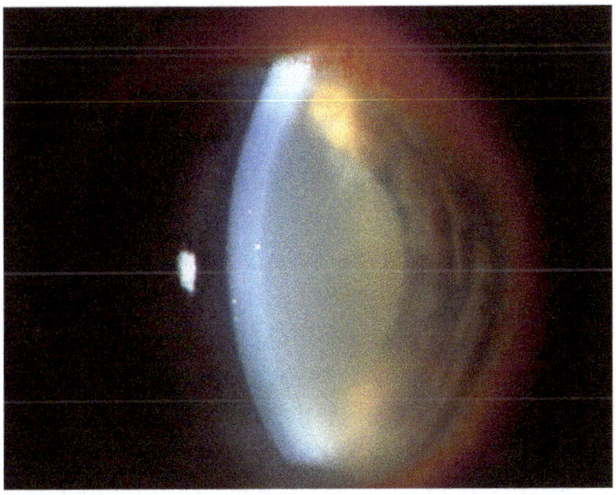

Fig. 6.11 Increase in IOP due to an overload of lens proteins in phacolysis

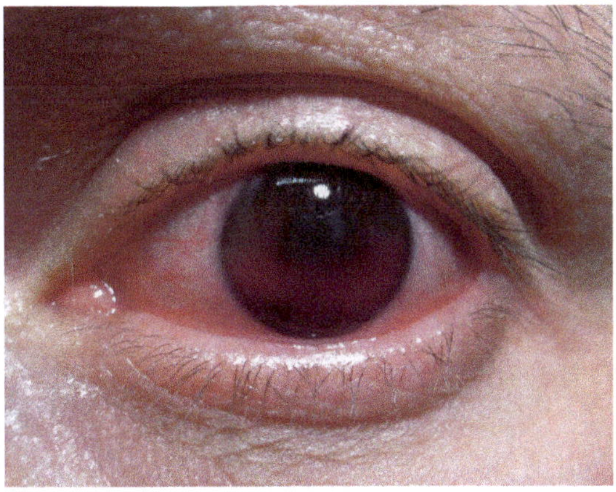

Fig. 6.12 Fresh hyphema after blunt trauma increasing the IOP due to compromising the outflow. Gonioscopy can be performed a week after resorption of the hyphema

cells do not have any color; their hemoglobin is lost over time.

6.2.1.5 Inflammatory Cells

Etiology/pathomechanisms: Inflammatory cells, fibrin and debris will obstruct the trabecular meshwork in uveitis due to juvenile idiopathic arthritis, HLA-B27-associated arthropathies (Fig. 6.13), Fuchs' uveitis, Posner-Schlossman syndrome (glaucomatous-cyclitic crisis), infections with herpes or zoster virus, syphilis, sarcoidosis (Figs. 6.14 and 6.15), tuberculosis, Vogt-Koyanagi-Harada syndrome, pars planitis or Behçet's disease.

In Fuchs' uveitis the corneal endothelium shows typical star-like precipitates, and the stromal layer of the iris is atrophic, therefore

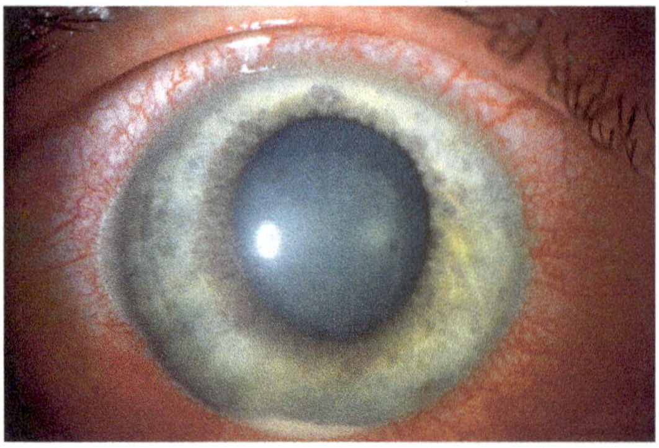

Fig. 6.13 Dense fibrin and a hypopyon in an eye with acute iridocyclitis (HLA B27-positive patient)

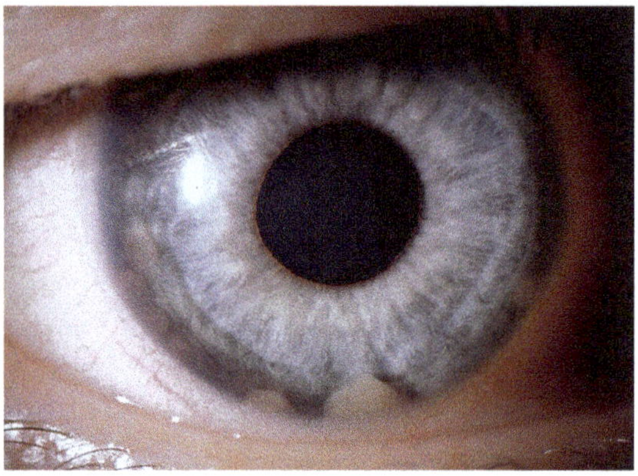

Fig. 6.14 Typical granulomatous nodules in the periphery of the iris, called Busacca nodules

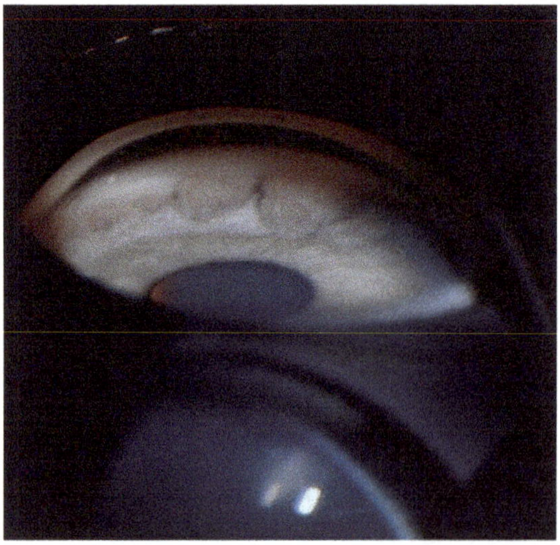

Fig. 6.15 Chamber angle of the same eye as shown in Fig. 6.14 with granulomatous nodules consisting of inflammatory cells

making the vessels more visible. During cataract or glaucoma surgery, when the IOP is very low for a short time, blood may come out of the vessels of the chamber angle (Amsler-Verrey sign). In herpetic trabeculitis the endothelial cells of the trabecular meshwork are swollen and the outflow resistance is very high. In Posner-Schlossman syndrome the pressure is even higher.

Note: Due to peripheral anterior synechiae or neovascularizations, a secondary angle-closure glaucoma may develop. Complete posterior synechia lead to an iris bombata with convex forward bowing of the iris and subsequently a secondary angle closure.

6.2.1.6 Tumor Cells

Etiology/pathomechanisms: Anterior segment tumors or disseminated tumor cells or tumor-related inflammatory cells may obstruct parts of the trabecular meshwork.

Chamber angle: Tumor masses or (mostly pigmented) tumor cells or inflammatory cells are found in the trabecular meshwork or the chamber angle.

6.2.1.7 After Ocular Trauma

Etiology/pathomechanisms: Blunt trauma may cause tears in all structures of the chamber angle including detachment of the ciliary body. Penetrating injuries may lead to severe changes of the structures due to scarring after inflammation. Chemical burns may destroy the endothelial cells of the trabecular meshwork. Some of the possible types of damage to structures of the chamber angle are illustrated in Fig. 6.16.

If the impact on the eye came from an orthograde direction, an iridodialysis or tears of the iris sphincter muscle are possible. In contrast, a lateral impact on the limbus will lead to a splitting inside the muscle parts of the ciliary muscle.

Injuries of the trabecular meshwork are not always visible. If the trabecular meshwork is torn, it can become detached from Schwalbe's ring and may form the shape of a roll. In the acute phase Schlemm's canal is filled with blood and shows a red line.

A very deep peripheral anterior chamber is a sign of zonular tears with (pseudo)phacodonesis (Fig. 6.17).

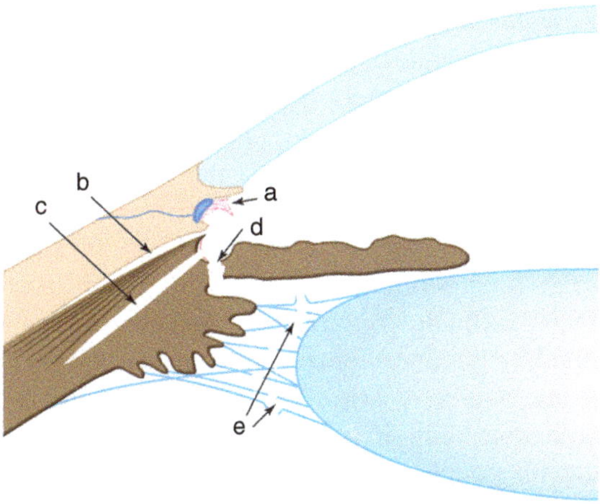

Fig. 6.16 Schematic drawing shows some of the possible types of damages to structures of the chamber angle: (*a*) tear of the trabecular meshwork, (*b*) detachment of the ciliary body (cyclodialysis), (*c*) tear between the longitudinal and radial fibers of the ciliary body (angle recession), (*d*) tear of the base of the iris (iridodialysis); (*e*) rupture of the zonules (zonulolysis)

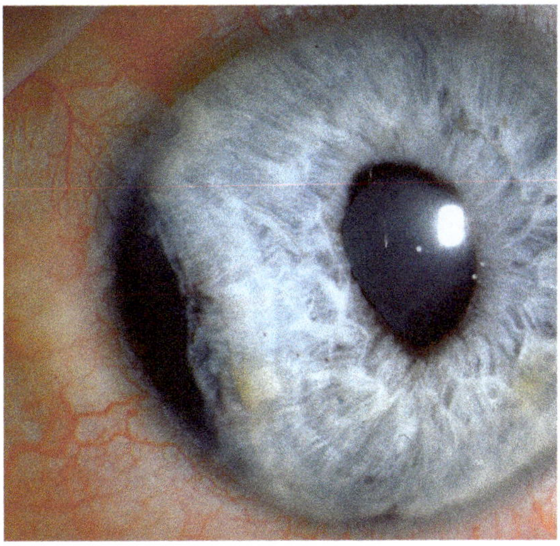

Fig. 6.18 Iridodialysis from 8 to 9:30 o'clock after severe blunt trauma. The ciliary processes are visible. The pigmented pupillary margin is lost from 8 to 9:30 o'clock

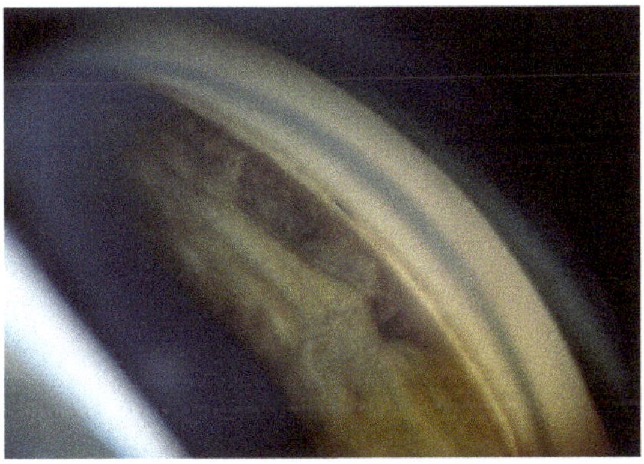

Fig. 6.17 Very deep peripheral anterior chamber due to tears of the peripheral iris and the zonular fiber after blunt trauma. There is an iridodialysis as a tear at the base of the iris and therefore the ciliary processes have become visible. The ciliary band, the white scleral spur and the trabecular meshwork (pigmentation +2) can be identified

The iris sphincter muscle may rupture partially or completely (fixed, wide pupil). You can find radial tears of the pupillary margin. If the iris dilator muscle is injured, a peripheral tear of the iris base will occur (iridodialysis; Fig. 6.18) and the pupil will no longer be round. In case of an iridodialysis you get a view into the posterior chamber to the ciliary processes gonioscopically.

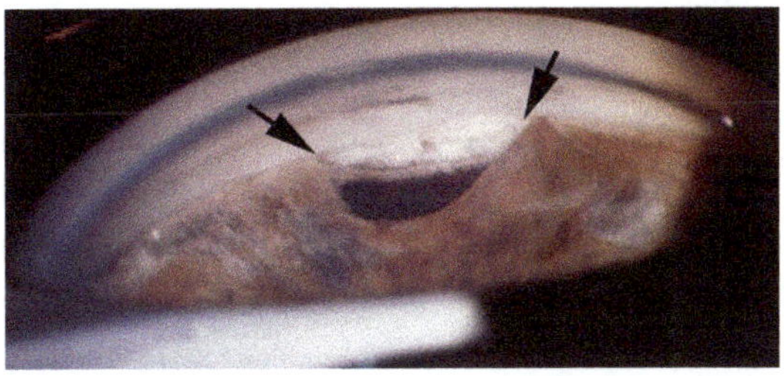

Fig. 6.19 Detachment of the ciliary body with visible white sclera (cyclodialysis, *between the arrows*), tear of the base of the iris with peripheral coloboma (iridodialysis) and peripheral anterior synechia close to the traumatic changes of the ciliary body and iris

Even parts of the ciliary muscle (between the longitudinal and radial parts, i.e. angle recession) tear or the ciliary body can become detached from the scleral spur (cyclodialysis; Fig. 6.19). In case of a cyclodialysis a cleft with the white sclera, spotted with some pigment, can be found gonioscopically.

Blood (hyphema) may be found if vessels are injured. Bleeding from a torn ciliary body is more common than from a torn trabecular meshwork. AS-OCT and/or UBM may help arrive at the proper diagnoses.

The lens might be dislocated and subluxated due to tears of the zonula fibers. Then you may find a larger cleft between the iris and the lens

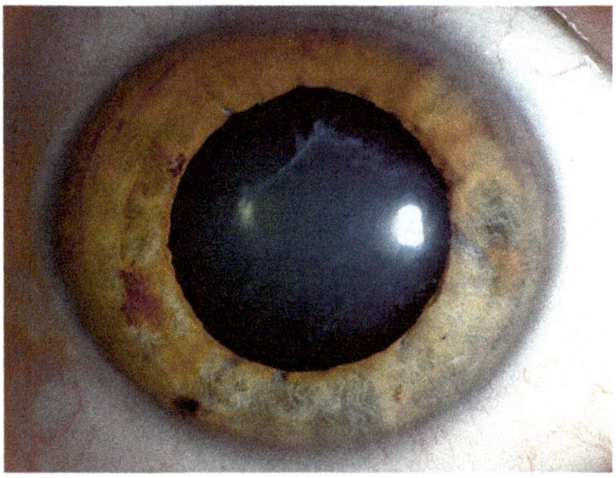

Fig. 6.20 Blunt trauma with subluxation of the lens posteriorly. Note the small radial tears in the pupillary margin of this fixed pupil

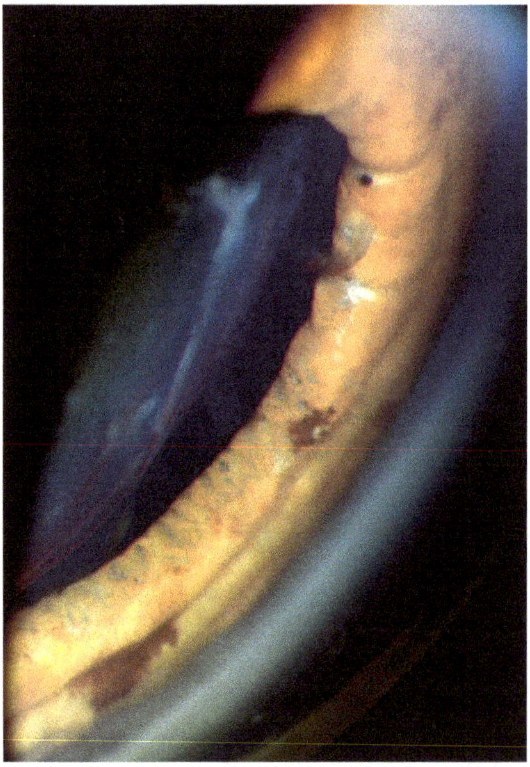

Fig. 6.21 There is a cleft between the lens surface and the iris, partially filled with vitreous

surface (possibly with vitreous between) and a very deep or closed angle (Figs. 6.20 and 6.21).

Do not overlook foreign bodies in the chamber angle. Sometimes they are covered by blood, so repeat the examination or order a plain radiography or CT.

Note: Due to peripheral anterior synechiae, a secondary angle-closed glaucoma may develop. The IOP may increase immediately after trauma due to an overload of the trabecular meshwork with blood cells, debris or pigment, but may also occur months or years later due to scarring or degenerative processes. The possibility of a steroid response can make trauma diagnosis even more difficult. Appropriate documentation is highly recommended and may be very helpful if a law suit may arise. Blood may obscure the structures until it is resorbed, after which the chamber angles of the two eyes can be compared to find differences. More severe injuries lead to a higher probability of posttraumatic glaucoma. Detachment of the ciliary body will decrease the IOP by increasing the uveoscleral outflow.

Don't mix up: recession (deepening) with recess (angle).

6.2.2 Open-Angle Glaucoma Caused by Extraocular Diseases

Etiology/pathomechanisms: Increased pressure in the episcleral venous system and the venous system of the orbit increases the outflow resistance. Reasons can be arteriovenous fistulae (too high pressure in the venous system due to an arterial shunt; Fig. 6.22), cavernous sinus thrombosis and obstructions of major veins (vena cava, jugular or pulmonary vein), Sturge-Weber

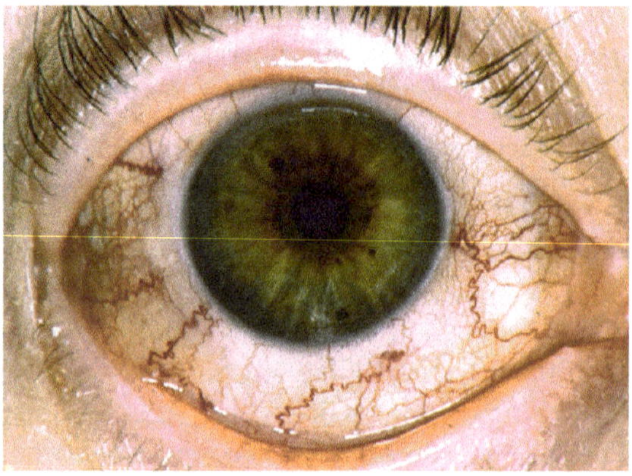

Fig. 6.22 An eye with engorgement of the conjunctival and scleral vessels due to a cavernous sinus thrombosis. The sound of pulsation may be heard through a stethoscope placed on the closed lids

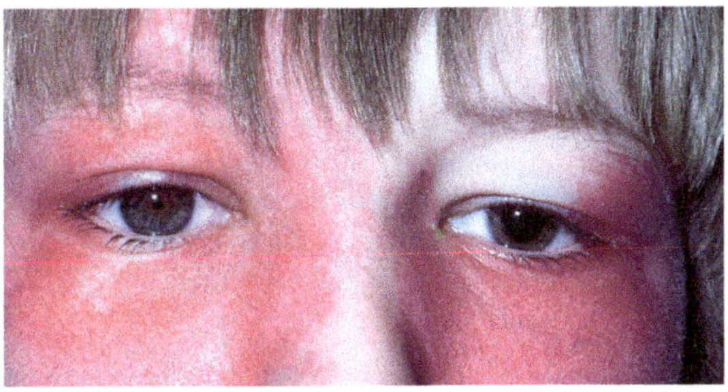

Fig. 6.23 Young patient with Sturge-Weber syndrome and glaucoma in his right eye, and a typical port wine stain of the skin of the face due to an overabundance of capillaries

syndrome (phacomatosis, encephalotrigeminal angiomatosis) with hemangioma (Fig. 6.23), orbital tumors with venous obstructions, endocrine orbitopathy with increased tissue tension in the orbit or changes of the conjunctival and scleral veins due to chemical burns or radiotherapy.

Chamber angle: Visible "red" Schlemm's canal shining through the trabecular meshwork, dilated episcleral veins.

6.2.3 Iatrogenic Open-Angle Glaucoma

6.2.3.1 Corticosteroid Treatment

Etiology/pathomechanisms: Steroids change the extracellular matrix of the trabecular meshwork after intravitreal administration. This may occur after more than 3–4 weeks topical administration or after months of systemic administration. Individuals with mutations of the positive trabecular meshwork glucocorticoid response (TIGR) gene or the myocilin gene are predisposed, as are myopic patients or patients with primary OAG.

Structures of the chamber angle: Regular.

Note: In about 6% of steroid responders, these changes of the meshwork are irreversible despite stopping the steroids.

6.2.3.2 Laser or Ocular Surgery

Etiology/pathomechanisms: Destruction of ocular tissue and release of inflammatory cells or debris:

- After argon laser trabeculoplasty, if the laser is applied with too high energy.

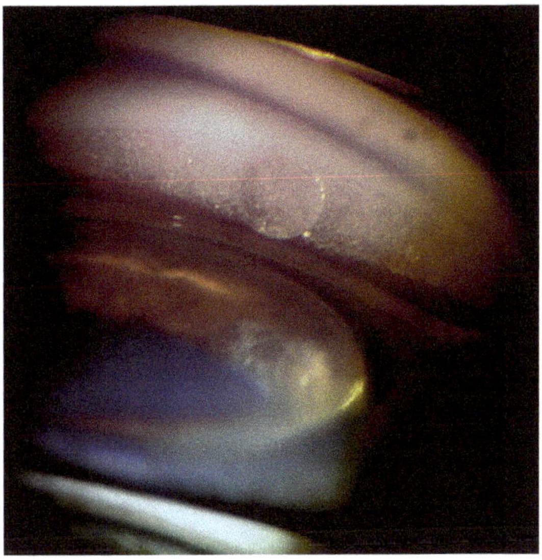

Fig. 6.24 Thousands of tiny silicone bubbles and one big bubble are present in the superior part of the chamber angle

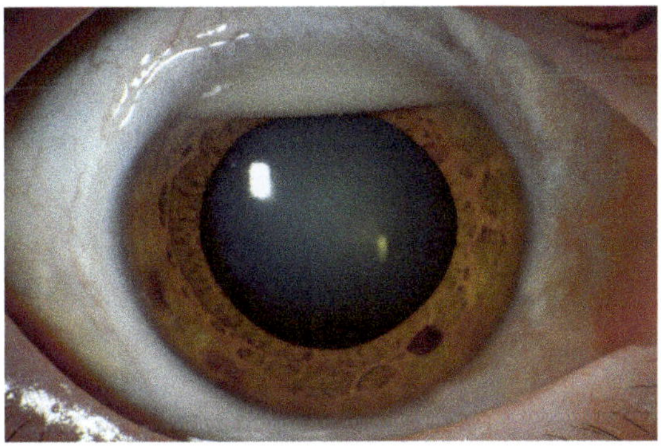

Fig. 6.25 An inverse "hypopyon" in the superior part of the chamber angle formed by emulsified silicone oil

- After Nd:YAG laser iridotomy, if the released pigment or tissue debris overloads the trabecular meshwork.
- After cataract surgery, if lens particles or remaining ocular viscoelastic device occlude the trabecular meshwork or toxic substances (toxic anterior segment syndrome) destroy the endothelial meshwork cells.
- After vitreoretinal surgery, if emulsified silicone oil is phagocytosed by the endothelial cells of the trabecular meshwork or has accumulated (Figs. 6.24 and 6.25)

Chamber angle, iris and lens: Changes due to cause. Emulsified silicone oil is always in the superior part of the open chamber angle, pigment (spotted) and debris in the inferior half.

Bibliography

Alward WL, Longmuir RA (2008) Color atlas of gonioscopy, 2nd edn. American Academy of Ophthalmology, San Francisco

Aptel F, Beccat S, Fortoul V, Denis P (2011) Biometric analysis of pigment dispersion syndrome using anterior segment optical coherence tomography. Ophthalmology 118:1563–1570

European Glaucoma Society (2008) Terminology and guidelines for glaucoma, 3rd edn. European Glaucoma Society/Dogma, Savona, Italy

Kersey JP, Broadway DC (2006) Corticosteroid-induced glaucoma: a review of the literature. Eye 20:407–416

Krieglstein GK, Kirchhof B (1994) Das Kammerwinkeltrauma. Z prakt Augenheilkd 15:15–25

Laemmer R, Mardin CY, Juenemann AG (2008) Visualization of changes of the iris configuration after peripheral laser iridotomy in primary melanin dispersion syndrome using optical coherence tomography. J Glaucoma 17:569–570

Quigley HA (2011) Glaucoma. Lancet 377:1367–1377

Schlötzer-Schrehardt U, Naumann GOH (2008) Morphology of exfoliation syndrome. In: Hollo G, Konstas AG (eds) Exfoliation syndrome and exfoliative glaucoma. Editrice Dogma, Savona, pp 33–44

7 Angle Closure and Glaucoma

7.1 The Chamber Angle in Primary Angle-Closure Disease

Considering primary open-angle glaucoma, the main resistance to outflow is in the cribriform layer (i.e. inner wall of Schlemm's canal) of the trabecular meshwork that leads to changes of the optic disc and the retinal nerve fiber layer (RNFL). In primary angle-closure disease, different amounts of iris tissue form contacts with the – originally intact and regular – trabecular meshwork, mainly as a result of forward bowing of the iris due to pupillary block (Figs. 7.1, 7.2, and 7.3). This iridotrabecular contact (ITC) is a totally different cause of glaucoma. And the initial therapy is significantly different between an open-angle glaucoma and closed-angle situation. Take care to distinguish between these two different entities!

7.1.1 Risk Factors

Risk factors for developing an angle closure may be changes in the anatomy of the eye, e.g. short eyes (hyperopic due to short axial length, nanophthalmus), shallow anterior chamber, lens with increased volume and/or vault (age, cataract; Fig. 7.4) or in spheroid shape (Weill-Marchesani syndrome) in combination with dilated pupils (e.g. on scotopic illumination). Specific ethnic groups (Inuit, East Asians) and women suffer more often from angle-closure disease.

Primary angle-closure disease seems to be a complex of mechanisms because of additional dynamic, physiological factors, such as choroidal expansion and/or thickness and iris volume changes when the pupil is dilated.

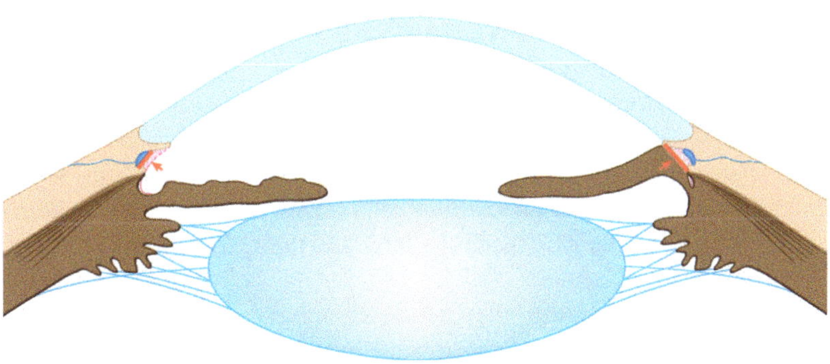

Fig. 7.1 Schematic drawing of the anterior chamber showing the main difference between open-angle (*left*) and angle-closure (*right*) diseases. The *red blocks* are the pathological sites

C. Faschinger, A. Hommer, *Gonioscopy*,
DOI 10.1007/978-3-642-28610-0_7, © Springer-Verlag Berlin Heidelberg 2012

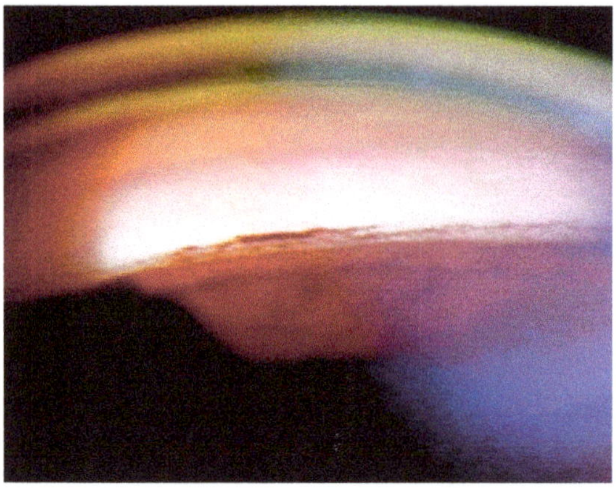

Fig. 7.2 A chamber angle in an eye with angle closure due to appositions (ITC) before indentation gonioscopy. Only a short line of pigment is visible

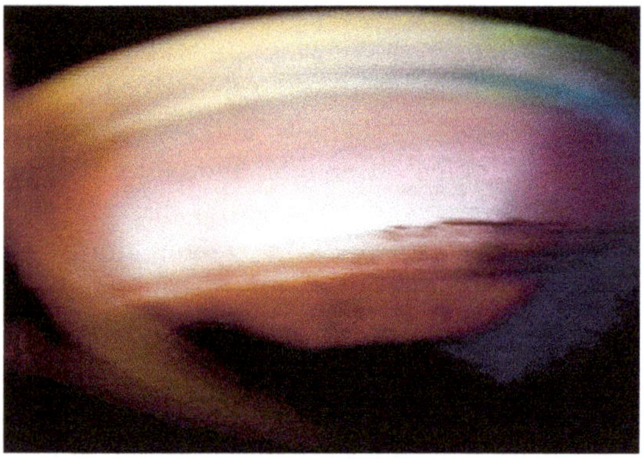

Fig. 7.3 During indentation gonioscopy of the same eye as in Fig. 7.2, the scleral spur, the pigmented trabecular meshwork (grade +2 to +3), Schwalbe's ring and some pigment anterior to Schwalbe's ring have become visible (Courtesy G. Megevand-Sunarevic)

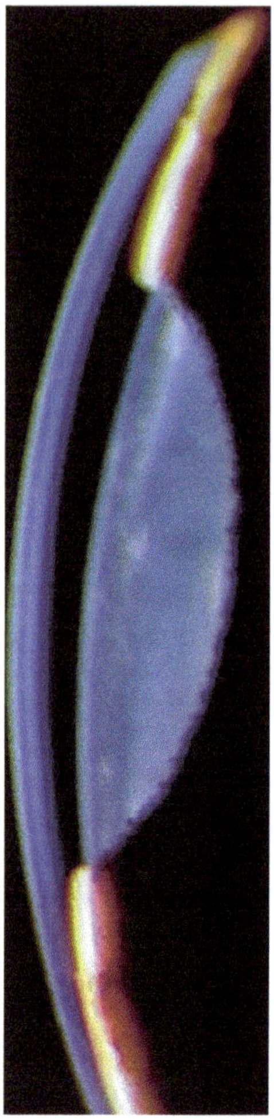

Fig. 7.4 Shallow central anterior chamber in an eye with a thickened lens due to cataract. A pupillary block and subsequent angle closure are highly probable

7.1.2 Terminology and Classification of Morphological and Functional Changes

- *Primary angle-closure suspect (PACS)*: The chamber angle shows appositions or ITC over 270° or more. The IOP, the disc/RNFL and the visual field are normal.
- *Primary angle closure (PAC)*: The chamber angle shows ITC or/and peripheral anterior synechiae. The IOP is >21 mmHg, the disc/RNFL and the visual field are normal. Appositions usually start in the recess at the iris root ("creeping angle closure", "B-type", mostly superior) or ITCs leave the recess open, but close the angle beyond ("S-type", mostly inferior). This indicates, that the insertion of the inferior iris is more posterior. Two-thirds of patients who have previously experienced an acute angle-closure attack (AAC) show no signs of glaucomatous changes in their disc or visual field, but their iris shows a torque structure and they have pigment depositions on the trabecular meshwork. They are also diagnosed as having PAC.
- *Primary angle-closure glaucoma (PACG)*: The chamber angle shows ITC or/and peripheral anterior synechiae. The IOP is >21 mmHg, the disc

Table 7.1 Classification of angle-closure diseases

Terminology	ITC, appositions >270°	Synechiae	IOP (mmHg)	Disc, visual field
PAC suspect	+	–	<21	Normal
PAC	+	±	>21	Normal
PACG	+	±	>21	Pathological

and the visual field are pathological (increased cup/disc ratio and visual field defect).

- *Acute angle closure (attack)* (*AAC*): Rapid closure of (nearly) the complete circumference of the chamber angle with very high IOP and severe symptoms and signs.

An appropriate diagnosis is only possible by careful indentation/dynamic gonioscopy with a small and dim slit beam in a dark room. An ITC will open during indentation; a synechia will remain (see Chap. 2, Sect. 2.3).

Note: Only a minority of patients with angle closure (PACS, PAC, PACG) report symptoms such as intermittent pain (differential diagnosis is migraine) or colored rings when looking into a light source. The majority show no symptoms, except in very severe glaucomatous damage.

A system of classification of angle-closure diseases is shown in Table 7.1.

7.1.3 Terms

7.1.3.1 "Occludable" Angle?

Per se any angle is occludable. Even a wide-open angle might become occluded over time by the increasing volume of a lens with cataract. However, an a priori narrow angle will become occluded with a much higher probability. A prophylactic iridotomy is generally performed in the second eye of patients with an AAC in the first eye or in eyes with chamber angles graded Shaffer 1 which need regular mydriasis due to diabetic retinopathy or in those with peripheral retinal degeneration.

It is necessary to differentiate between a closed angle (which is either reversibly closed by ITC or irreversible closed by synechiae) and an open angle *at the time of examination*.

Angles graded 1 (gonioscopically Shaffer or slit lamp van Herick) have a high probability of becoming "occluded" or closed in the future, but not necessarily all of them. In fact, the probability is about 1:10 in those eyes in which the volume of the iris increases instead of decreases with pupillary dilation.

In population survey studies the definition of an "occludable" angle is an angle in which only 90° or less of the functional, posterior trabecular meshwork is visible.

7.1.3.2 "Narrow"-Angle Glaucoma

This term derives from the days before indentation gonioscopy was known, and should be avoided. The angle is either open or closed. "Narrow" is a qualitative term and does not imply occludable or not occludable. There are conditions of the eyes with primary open-angle glaucoma in which the chambers are narrowed without any ITC or synechiae as a result of an increase in the lens volume. However, such a condition remains an open-angle glaucoma with a chamber angle graded 1 or 2 (Shaffer) and the main outflow resistance is in the cribriform trabecular meshwork. Additional pupillary block may develop, leading to further forward bowing of the iris, ITC or synechiae, and therefore to a "secondary" angle-closure glaucoma.

7.1.3.3 "Acute Angle-Closure" Glaucoma

An acute attack with closure of almost the total circumference of the angle and high IOP not necessarily is leading to an optic neuropathy, i.e. glaucoma per se. The optic disc may sustain no damage in the majority of cases with a single event. A single attack does not lead to progressive disease, and therefore it is "per definition" no glaucoma.

7.1.4 Classification of the Causes of Angle Closure

Four levels may help classify the causes of angle-closure (glaucoma).

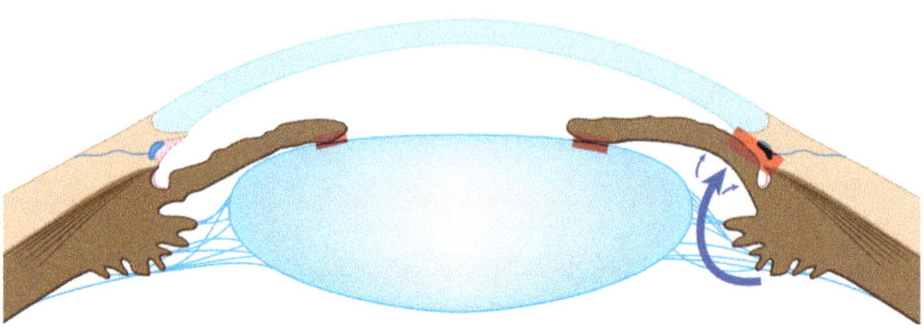

Fig. 7.5 Schematic drawing showing a pupillary block in a mid–wide pupil and the subsequent forward bowing of the iris and closure of the chamber angle

7.1.4.1 Level 1: Iris and Pupillary Block

The competing forces of the iris muscles, the sphincter and dilator of the pupil, create a vector force at the margin of the pupil that is directed posteriorly onto the anterior surface of the lens. This occurs when the pupil is of medium width. Remember that pseudoexfoliation material is rubbed off the surface of the lens in the mid-periphery of the lens surface giving the appearance of a doughnut.

The pupillary margin blocks the flow of the aqueous humor from the posterior to the anterior chamber. Subsequently the iris, predominantly in the peripheral, thinner part will bow forward. The lens acts like a ball valve and closes the flow of the aqueous humor through the pupil. Iris tissue will form contacts with the trabecular meshwork or Schwalbe's ring (ITC). Some of the contacts will release by themselves (pupil constricts, "intermittent" angle closure), and some will change to peripheral anterior synechiae (Fig. 7.5).

Note: only a minority of patients experience subjective symptoms such as pain, red eye or halos when looking into light sources. The majority show no symptoms.

If posterior synechiae (i.e. between iris and lens) have led to a forward bowing of the iris, we speak about "iris bombata" or "iris bombé".

Predisposing factors for a pupillary block in an anatomically predisposed eye are, for example: diagnostic mydriasis, watching TV or movies in a cinema with dim light, emotional situations with high adrenergic output, drugs (e.g. antidepressant serotonin uptake inhibitors).

New Insights

Why does not everybody with a narrow angle develop ITC or synechiae or develop an angle closure? "The iris is like a sponge", wrote Quigley et al. in 2000. They observed the dynamics of the iris change during dilation in the dark and constriction in bright light by means of AC-OCT and found that the iris usually gets smaller upon dilation due to volume loss and enlarges as the pupil narrows. The iris acts like a sponge—water moves in and out of it. People with narrow angles loose less iris volume upon dilation.

7.1.4.2 Level 2: Ciliary Body: Plateau Iris

Plateau iris configuration is a gonioscopic finding, where at least one of the following items should be determined (Fig. 7.6)

- Thick peripheral iris roll.
- Anterior insertion of the iris (anterior to the scleral spur).
- Anterior insertion and rotation of the ciliary body so that the ciliary processes are visible on gonioscopy. There is no or almost no ciliary sulcus. UBM and/or AS-OCT provide an additional insight into the anatomical structures behind the iris.
- Very steep peripheral iris with normal depth of the anterior chamber centrally. The angle is narrow ($<10°$) or closed for at least 180°. The central iris is flat (Fig. 7.7).
- "Double hump sign" or "sinus wave sign" in indentation gonioscopy. A peripheral hump of the iris is seen by the anteriorly rotated ciliary body, and a more centrally located second hump of the iris is formed by the shoulder of the lens (Fig. 7.8).

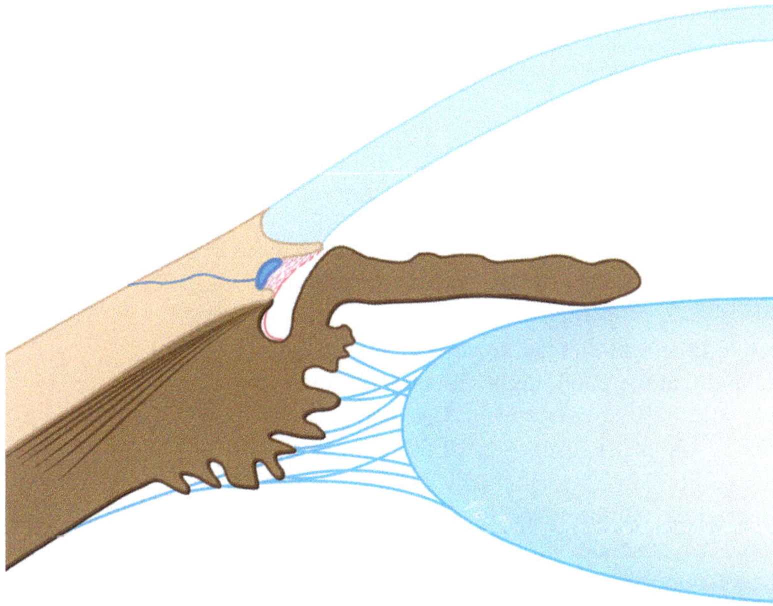

Fig. 7.6 Schematic drawing showing four signs characteristic of a plateau iris configuration: a thick peripheral iris roll, an anterior insertion of the iris, an anterior rotation of the ciliary body, a very steep peripheral iris and a flat central iris with an almost normal depth of the anterior chamber

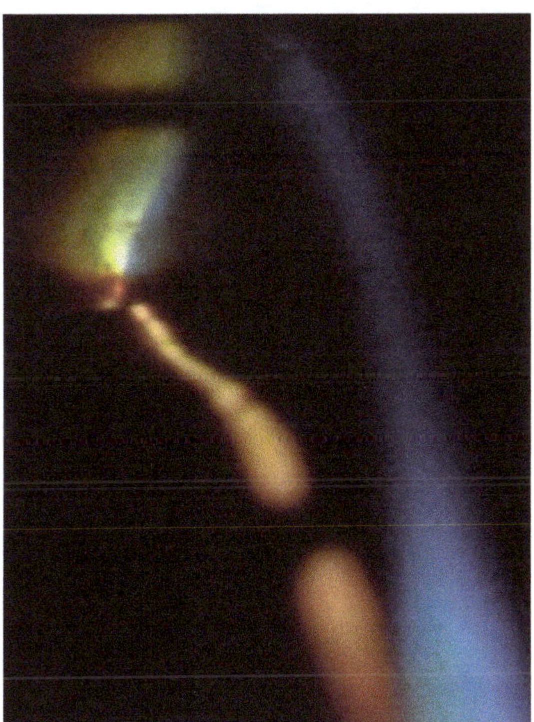

Fig. 7.7 Flat iris with normal depth of the anterior chamber, but very steep drop-off of the iris into the chamber angle. The scleral spur and a heavily pigmented trabecular meshwork are visible

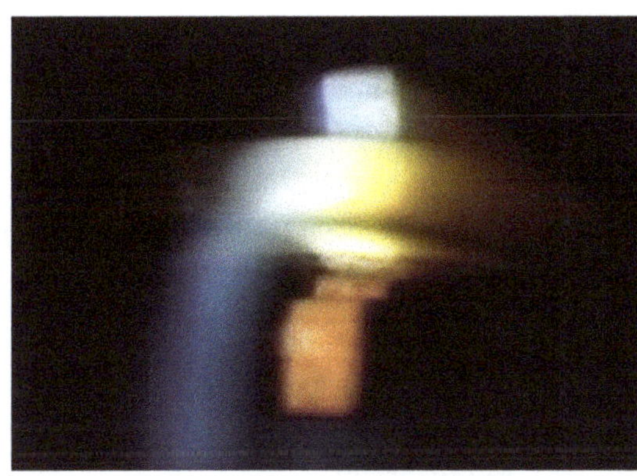

Fig. 7.8 "Double hump sign" during indentation gonioscopy. The peripheral hump is from the anteriorly rotated ciliary body, and the more central hump from the shoulder of the lens

To release the pupillary block a peripheral iridotomy is recommended. The majority will be healed.

In eyes without pupillary block and/or iris tissue very close to the trabecular meshwork, an increase in the IOP will result after dilation of the pupil despite a patent iridotomy and the diagnosis will change to *plateau iris syndrome*. This will lead to peripheral anterior synechiae and closure of the angle. Sometimes chronic use of pilocarpine 1–0.1% is indicated.

The next step in treatment would be an argon laser peripheral iridoplasty. Argon laser burns are placed circumferentially on the peripheral parts of the iris to shrink the tissue and flatten the periphery of the iris. The pupil is constricted with pilocarpine 1% preoperatively. Inform the patient before treatment that the procedure may be painful and that the pupil might remain larger than it was before the laser treatment. Use a contact lens (Wise, Abraham), a spot size of 500 μm, a pulse duration of 0.2–0.5 s, an energy of 200–400 mW (depending on the color of the iris), and five burns per quadrant. Postoperatively nonsteroidal antiinflammatory eye drops are given (see Chap. 9, Sect. 9.1.3)

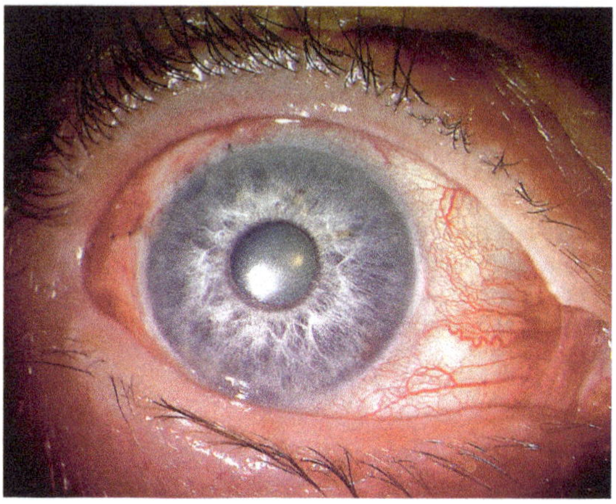

Fig. 7.9 Eye on the first day after filtration surgery. The anterior chamber is very shallow centrally and almost gone in the periphery. The peripheral iridectomy is patent, and running limbal suture of conjunctiva/Tenon's capsule is visible (IOP 22 mmHg)

7.1.4.3 Level 3: Lens

An increase in the thickness of the lens (intumescent cataract, nuclear cataract, "phacomorphic" glaucoma) or a change in the position of the lens (subluxation after trauma or in pseudoexfoliation due to weak zonules) may lead to a forward pushing of the iris and closure of the chamber angle. Treatment is cataract surgery, which is not always simple in these eyes.

7.1.4.4 Level 4: Retrolenticular Aqueous Misdirection

This troublesome (for the patient as well as the surgeon) reaction of an eye after trabeculectomy or cataract surgery needs special care. It is also called "malignant glaucoma", but this term should be avoided so as not to upset or confuse the patient with the association to cancer.

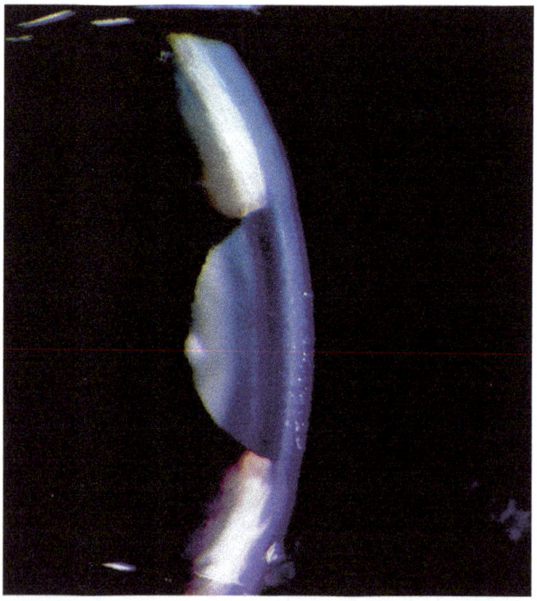

Fig. 7.10 Same eye as shown in Fig. 7.9 (slit beam examination) with a very shallow anterior chamber, but without the lens touching the corneal endothelium

In an eye with a recent trabeculectomy, a very shallow anterior chamber despite an open iridectomy, no choroidal effusion and a relatively high IOP (between 15 and 20 mmHg or more; Figs. 7.9 and 7.10) should arouse the suspicion of aqueous misdirection. Usually eyes with a shallow anterior chamber postoperatively have a very low IOP (0–5 mmHg). The main reasons are a ciliolenticular block (Fig. 7.11) and an increase in volume in the choroids. A ciliolenticular block is a blockage between a thick, anterior rotated ciliary muscle and its processes and the equator of the lens, preventing the aqueous humor from flowing anteriorly.

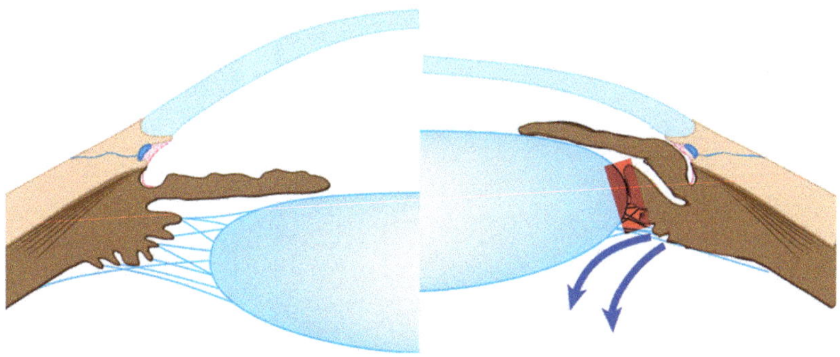

Fig. 7.11 Schematic drawing showing a regular, wide open chamber angle on the *left* and a ciliolenticular block on the *right*. The aqueous humor cannot pass between the ciliary body and its processes and the equator of the lens. Therefore, it is misdirected into the vitreous cavity shifting the iris–lens diaphragm forward

The aqueous humor is misdirected into the vitreous cavity, pushing the iris–lens diaphragm forward, inducing the angle closure.

The first aim is to relax the ciliary body by the application of anticholinergic drugs (atropine five times a day) and to stop further production of aqueous humor by the administration of carbonic anhydrase inhibitors intravenously and orally. Be patient! "Sit on your fingers"! It takes about 3 days for the anterior chamber to become deeper. Do not be tempted and do not try to fill the anterior chamber with viscoelastic agents. This will not work, and will probably end in disaster. The use of miotics such as pilocarpine will worsen the situation due to increased thickening and anterior rotation of the ciliary body.

If cornea–lens contact cannot be avoided or the IOP gets too high for a too long period, complete vitrectomy via the pars plana with disruption of the anterior hyaloid membrane combined with a tunneling might be indicated. The "tunnel" is made with the vitrectome from the posterior chamber, cutting the zonules and passing through the existing iridectomy or creating a new iridectomy into the anterior chamber, always in combination with a phacoemulsification. If the lens is not removed it would be damaged. Another treatment option might be a diode cyclophotocoagulation to shrink the ciliary body. UBM and/or AS-OCT may provide an overview of the anatomical situation.

This dreadful complication of aqueous misdirection occurs typically in very short eyes (axial length <21 mm) and higher hyperopics.

Note: Levels 1 and 2 are *bilateral* conditions (mostly) and may be managed by constriction of the pupil (e.g. with pilocarpine) while levels 3 and 4 are *asymmetrical* conditions and may be managed by dilation of the pupil (with atropine) and relaxation of the ciliary body.

7.1.5 Acute Angle Closure (Attack)

Rapid closure of (nearly) the complete circumference of the chamber angle leads to very high IOP and severe symptoms and signs.

Symptoms: Heavy pain in the orbit, nausea, vomiting, even pain (cramps) in the stomach. Visual acuity is decreased, possibly to perception only of hand movements or light. On palpation the globe feels hard like a stone.

Signs: The conjunctiva is red and the vessels are dilated (venous congestion). The cornea is thickened and hazy due to the fluid (aqueous humor) that is pressed into the corneal stroma and epithelium. The central anterior chamber is very shallow; the peripheral chamber absent. The pupil is mid-dilated and does not react to light (Figs. 7.12, 7.13, 7.14, and 7.15).

The signs are so characteristic that gonioscopy in the acute phase does not provide any additional information. After lowering the IOP by systemic and local drugs a YAG iridotomy is highly indicated.

But: Check the second eye by gonioscopy, preferably indentation gonioscopy! You will almost always find a narrow, occludable or partially

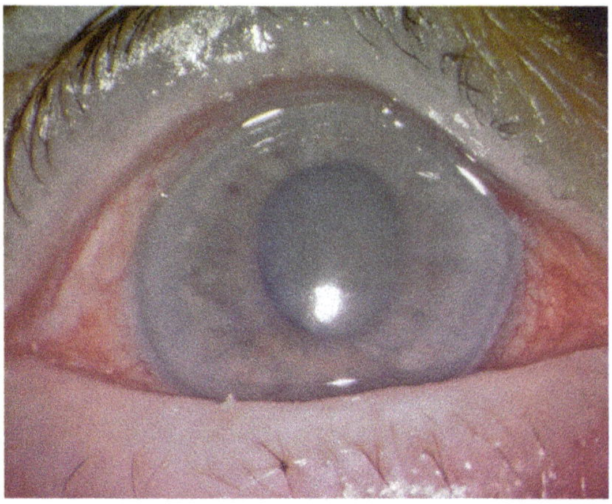

Fig. 7.12 Acute angle-closure attack with an IOP of 55 mmHg showing dilated conjunctival vessels, a hazy cornea, and a mid-wide pupil with hardly any light reaction

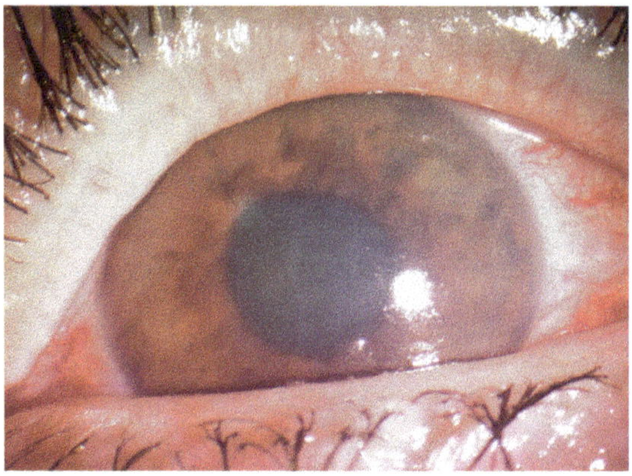

Fig. 7.14 Acute angle-closure attack with an IOP of 60 mmHg showing a thick brown iris, a mid–wide pupil, and a hazy cornea

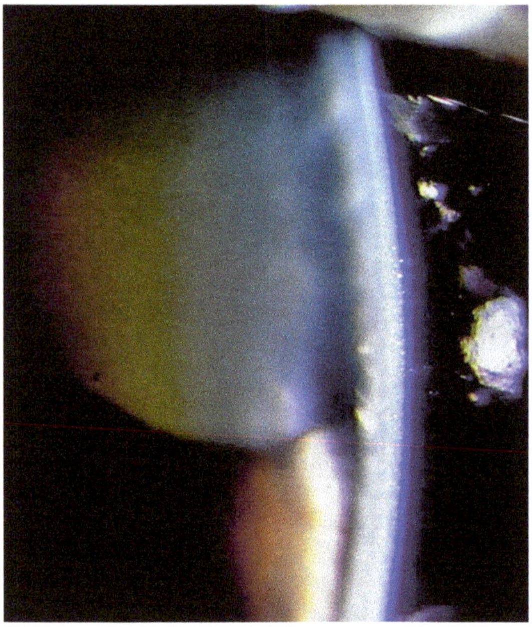

Fig. 7.13 Thick cornea due to edema and thick lens with yellow cataract. The axial length is 19.58 mm (same eye as shown Fig. 7.13)

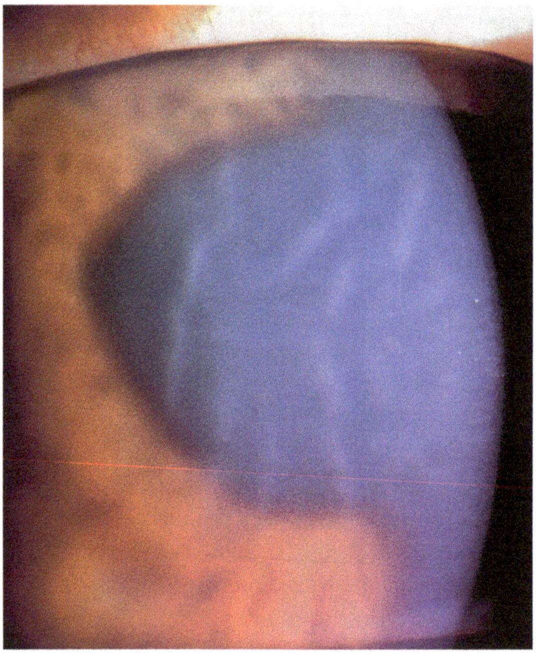

Fig. 7.15 Corneal edema and folds due to very high IOP (same eye as shown in Fig. 7.15)

occluded angle, without or with appositions or ITCs. Do not forget to perform a prophylactic iridotomy in this eye, too!

And: Find out if the pupil was dilated by drops, if drugs were taken (see Chap. 11), what kind of emotions the patient was experiencing, and what kind of activities (TV, reading, cinema) the patient was engaged in before the onset of the attack. The answers will give you more insight.

In almost all patients an acute angle closure is a unique experience, and astonishingly leads to only minor loss of visual function. Rarely will the optic disc become pale. Disc edema and splinter hemorrhages are seldom seen during the acute angle closure but if they do occur rarely lead to glaucomatous cupping.

As the configuration of the chamber angle is hereditary in about 60% of individuals, relatives should have their chamber angle checked for signs of angle closure.

Therapy: Lowering of the IOP by intravenous or oral (if patient is not vomiting) administration of a carbonic anhydrase inhibitor (acetazolamide), but first ask about allergy to sulfonamides. Topically administered carbonic anhydrase inhibitors are not indicated. Timolol 0.5% topically will also lower the pressure. Only if the pupillary reaction is positive (iris sphincter no longer ischemic) is pilocarpine indicated. The idea is to pull the peripheral iris out of the angle to open appositions. Give 2% pilocarpine drops three times every 10 min. Not more often, because pilocarpine as a parasympathomimetic drug constricts not only the pupil, but also the ciliary body, pushing the thickened muscle forward, closing the angle even more! The formerly used "pilo-bath", pilocarpine eye drops in a cup and the eye constantly in contact with the fluid, worsens angle closure and is absolutely obsolete.

Steroids topically are given to reduce the amount of adhesions of the iris to the trabecular meshwork. The use of 10% glycerol eye drops might clear up the cornea so that it becomes transparent enough for iridotomy.

7.1.6 Status Post-Acute Angle-Closure (Attack)

There are several signs showing that the eye has previously experienced an acute angle-closure: the iris is partially atrophic, the normally regular and radial structure of the iris is twisted (Fig. 7.16), the pupil is less reactive due to an ischemic lesion of the iris sphincter muscle, sometimes in combination with posterior synechiae, the lens shows small milky white spots beneath the anterior capsule (*Glaukomflecken*, Fig. 7.17), the endothelial cells may be compromised, and the chamber angle shows peripheral anterior synechiae on gonioscopy.

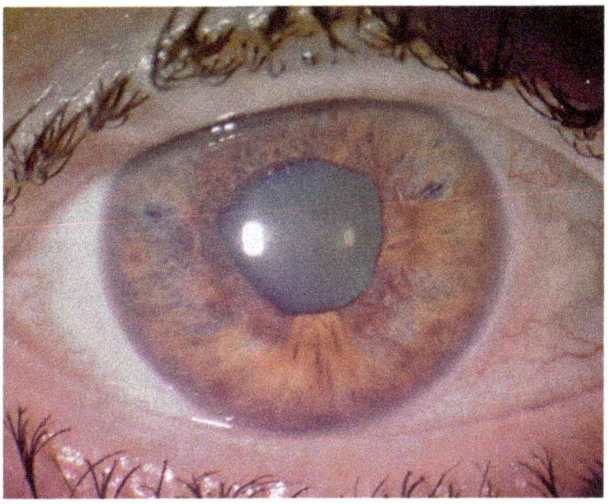

Fig. 7.16 The structure of the anterior layer of the iris is no longer radial; it is twisted and the tissue is partially atrophic. There are two open iridotomies, at 9:30 and 2:30 o'clock

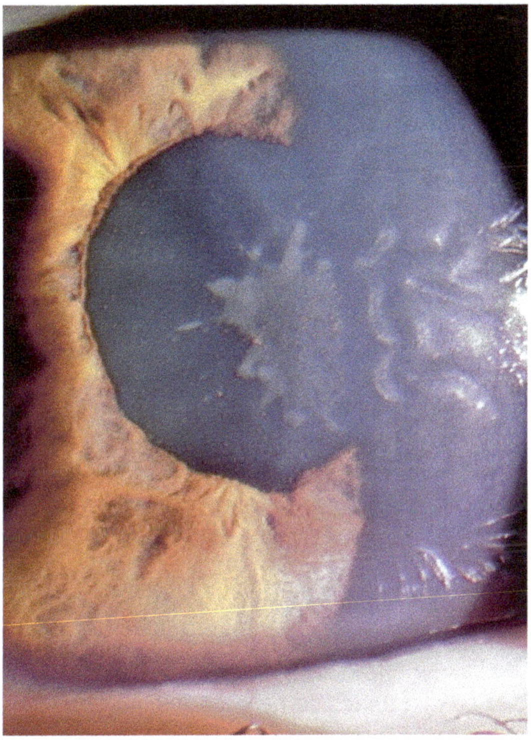

Fig. 7.17 *Glaukomflecken* ("spilt milk") sign of an acute angle-closure attack

The longer the closure lasts the higher the probability that the peripheral iris will remain in contact with the trabecular meshwork, forming spotted pigment deposits and peripheral anterior synechiae with functional damage to the trabecular meshwork.

7.1.7 Management of Angle-Closure Disease

Treatment is usually step-wise:

Start with a Nd:YAG peripheral iridotomy (LPI) or surgical iridectomy in eyes with more than 270° of appositions/ITC and normal IOP and normal disc/visual field. Such eyes are diagnosed as suspicious for primary angle closure. Add IOP-lowering eye drops in eyes with synechiae and IOP more than 21 mmHg. Such eyes are diagnosed as primary angle closure. If cataract is present, perform phacoemulsification. Argon Laser peripheral iridoplasty might be considered to stretch the peripheral iris tissue between the synechiae.

In eyes with loss of neuroretinal tissue and progressive visual field loss (primary angle-closure glaucoma), filtration surgery might be indicated. Be careful: "small eyes – big troubles" (P. Foster). They sometimes develop an aqueous misdirection ("malignant glaucoma"). Check the axial length and the scleral thickness before surgery. In some cases a surgical goniosynechialysis may be of benefit.

7.1.7.1 Nd:YAG Laser Peripheral Iridotomy (LPI), Iridectomy

Inform the patient about the intended treatment, about possible side effects and about the consequences of no treatment. It is important to bear in mind that iridotomy per se does not lower the IOP (sometimes, in contrast, it increases the pressure due to debris and pigment release); it only corrects a pupillary block.

Premedication with miotics will facilitate the perforation by unfolding the iris and reducing its thickness.

Look for an iris crypt so that as little debris as possible is released. The preferred position should be between 11 and 1 o'clock, covered by the upper lid, to avoid probable postoperative photic phenomena. A single hole of at least 200 μm in diameter is enough. You will see the gush of pigment pouring into the anterior chamber. This pigment can be found later in the inferior part of the chamber angle as pigmented spots.

If the iris is too thick to be perforated with the Nd:YAG laser only, you may pretreat the iris with an argon Laser. Or you can perform a surgical iridectomy via a corneal approach so as not to irritate the conjunctiva because filtration surgery will probably be needed later. This provides the benefit of deepening the anterior chamber with fluid or viscoelastics which releases all or a few anterior synechiae (goniosynechialysis). In addition, in surgical iridectomy the outflow facility of the trabecular meshwork will not be compromised by the presence of debris.

Note: Check the width of the chamber angle after 1 week: it should be wider after iridotomy. If this is not the case, think about cataract surgery in a quiet interval because of a phacomorphic component to the angle closure. The central depth of the anterior chamber will remain unchanged after iridotomy. The deepening of the peripheral anterior chamber has been shown in a prospective study evaluating UMB. The depth increased significantly in all four quadrants, e.g. in the superior quadrant from 3.59° preoperatively to 12.58° postoperatively.

7.2 The Chamber Angle in Secondary Angle Closure

There are no differences between secondary and primary angle closure in the aspect of the chamber angle; the only difference is in the causative event, which is either an ocular or a systemic disease. In gonioscopy parts of the peripheral iris or the complete peripheral iris are in contact with the trabecular meshwork, the anterior ciliary band or Schwalbe's ring, forming irido-trabecular appositions and/or peripheral anterior synechiae.

In some eyes a secondary angle closure may develop from a primary open angle. Since primary glaucoma is usually bilateral, an asymmetry in angle width, for example an open angle in one eye and a narrow or closed angle in the other eye, are predictive of some secondary mechanism (if the eyes are similar in refraction).

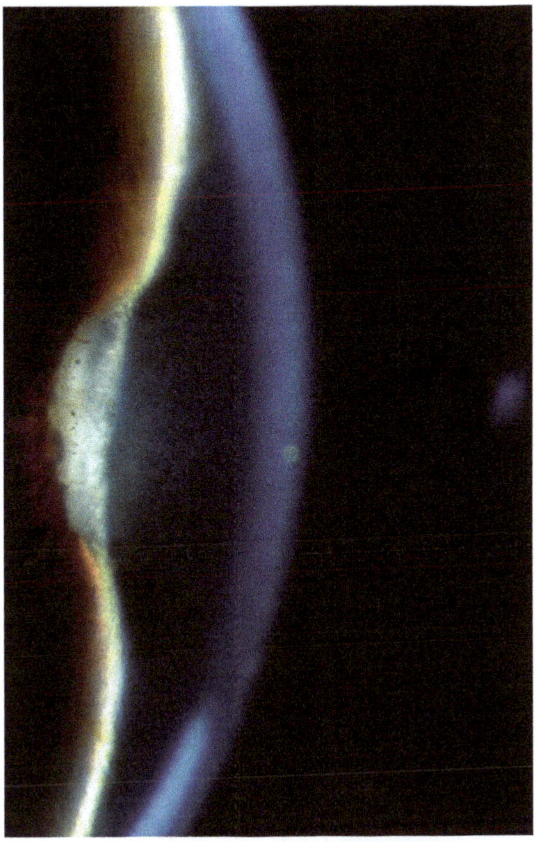

Fig. 7.18 Slitlamp photograph of an eye with iris bombata due to circular posterior synechiae with dense cataract, and a shallow peripheral chamber

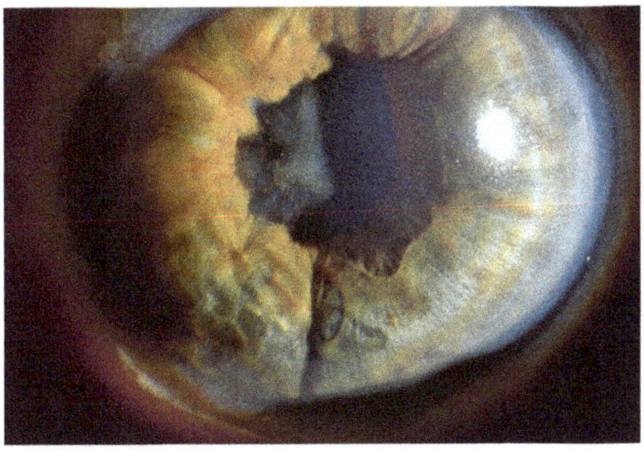

Fig. 7.19 Iris bombata in aphakia without an implant lens and circular synechiae with the anterior vitreous membrane in an eye with chronic uveitis

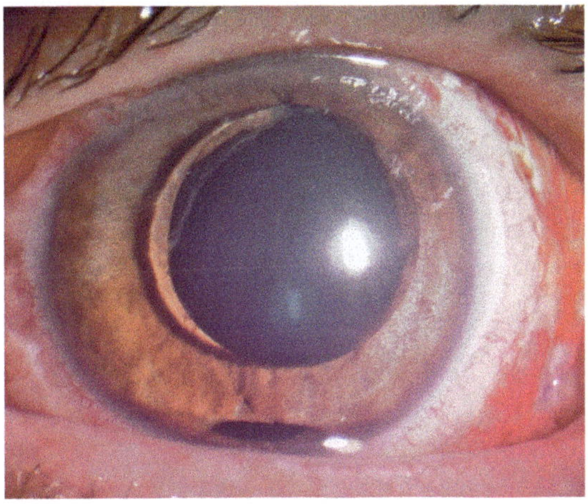

Fig. 7.20 Silicone oil blocking the pupil, but no angle-closure, due to an open inferior iridectomy

Remember: Perform gonioscopy under low light conditions!

7.2.1 Causes of Secondary Angle Closure

7.2.1.1 With Pupillary Block

In eyes with thick swollen lens (phacomorphic in advanced cataract), anterior lens dislocation due to weak zonules (pseudoexfoliation, trauma, Marfan syndrome, Weil-Marchesani syndrome).

In eyes with seclusion or occlusion of the pupillae with iris bombata (bombé) after inflammations due to circular posterior synechiae (Figs. 7.18 and 7.19).

In eyes with aphakia with:

- Prolapse of the vitreous into the pupil
- Prolapse of silicone oil into the pupil without an Ando iridectomy at 6 o'clock (Fig. 7.20)
- Aphakia and anterior chamber lens without a patent peripheral iridectomy (Fig. 7.21)
- Pseudophakia (refractive lenses) in phakic eyes without iridectomy

7.2.1.2 Without Pupillary Block, but with an Anterior Pulling Mechanism

In eyes with neovascular membranes. These consist not only of new vascular structures, but they also have proliferative fibrotic tissue. The vessels are

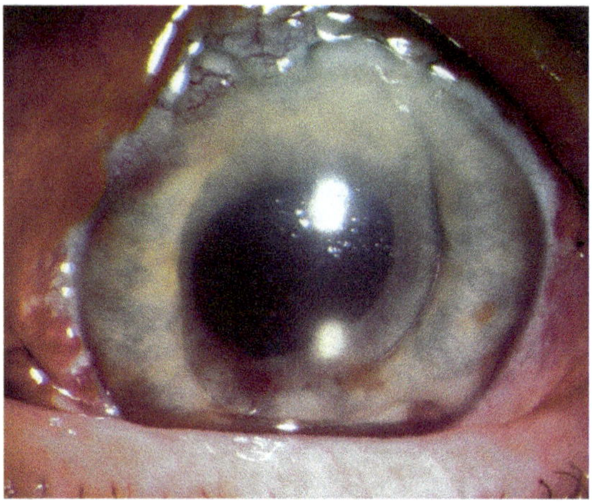

Fig. 7.21 Aphakia with anterior chamber lens (first post-operative day) with iridectomy not patent. The peripheral iris is bowed forward and pushed into the chamber angle

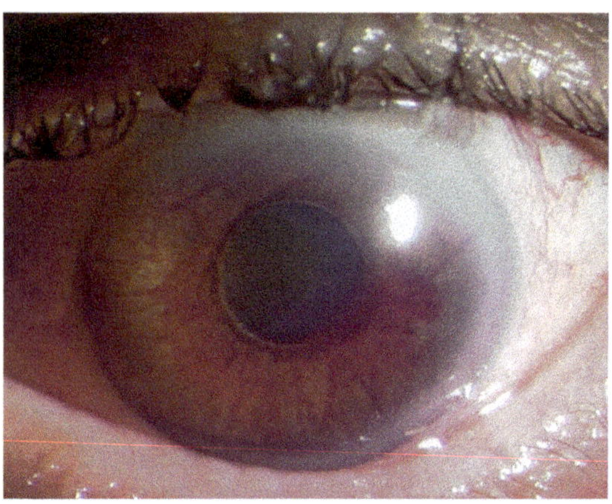

Fig. 7.22 Newly formed vessels on the anterior surface of the iris in a randomized pattern in an eye with a central venous thrombosis 6 months before

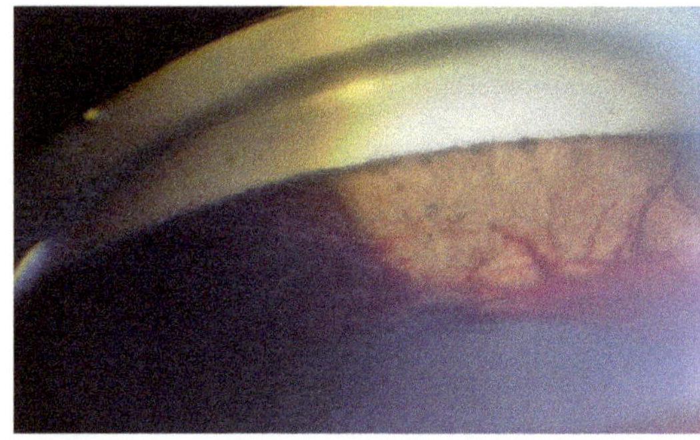

Fig. 7.23 Chamber angle of an eye with neovascularizations of the iris. There are no structures of the chamber angle visible; the angle is completely closed

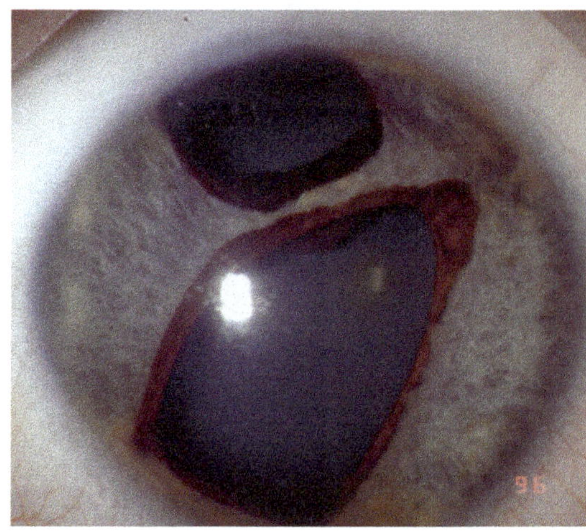

Fig. 7.24 Progressive essential iris atrophy due to proliferating endothelial cells showing ectopia of the pupil and a large hole in the iris at 12 o'clock

thinner than normal and they do not run in a radial or circumferential pattern (Fig. 7.22). Reasons can be proliferative diabetic retinopathy, central retinal venous occlusion, occlusion of the carotid, and rarely central retinal artery occlusion. The hypoxia induces an increase in the levels of growth factors. The fibrovascular tissue starts to proliferate at the pupillary margin of the iris, and grows towards the chamber angle (Fig. 7.23).

In eyes with iridocorneal endothelial syndrome (ICE), with progressive formation of endothelium and its basement membrane (Descemet's membrane). These structures have an abnormal tendency for proliferation, which pulls the iris into the chamber angle. The consequences are synechiae and distortion of the pupil (corectopia) and the formation of new pupils (polycoria) in the opposite direction to the pulling, with atrophy of iris tissue. The pulling mechanisms lead to an ectropium of the pigmented layer of the iris.

- Progressive (essential) iris atrophy: iris atrophy with marked corectopia, hole formations in the iris (pseudopolycoria), always unilateral (Figs. 7.24 and 7.25)
- Chandler syndrome: much less iris atrophy; ectropium uveae, corneal edema

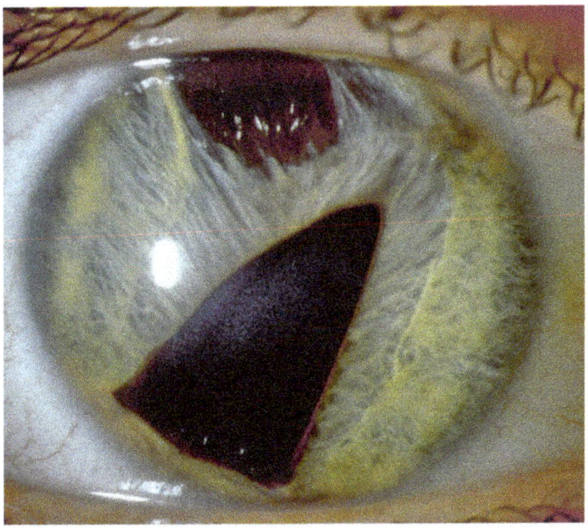

Fig. 7.25 The same eye as shown in Fig. 7.24 14 years later showing enlargement of the big hole and loss of pigmentary layer of the iris with a new large hole at 12 o'clock. The eye went blind after several operations

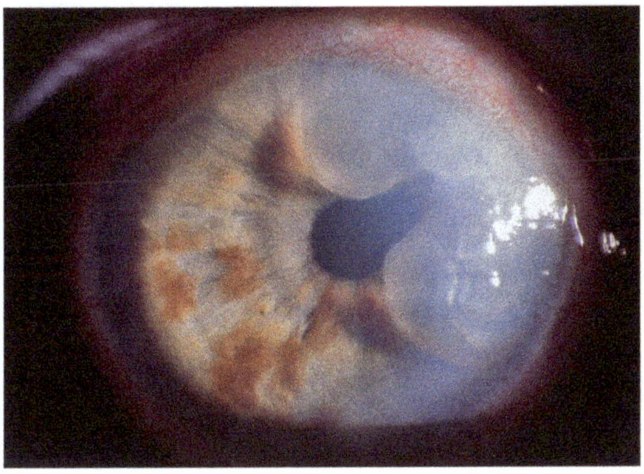

Fig. 7.26 Epithelial implant cysts from 12 to 5 o'clock in the chamber angle and the anterior chamber after extracapsular cataract extraction. The cysts are transparent and have grown slowly

- Iris-nevus syndrome (Cogan-Reese): peduncular nodules on the iris surface combined with iris atrophy

In eyes with epithelial ingrowth after penetrating globe injuries or surgery. The epithelium proliferates within a slowly increasing cyst (Fig. 7.26).

Following argon-laser trabeculoplasty, with the laser spots placed too close to the anterior ciliary band. The inflammation and the scars will lead to peripheral anterior synechiae.

In aniridia. The small amount of peripheral iris tissue tends to cover the trabecular meshwork.

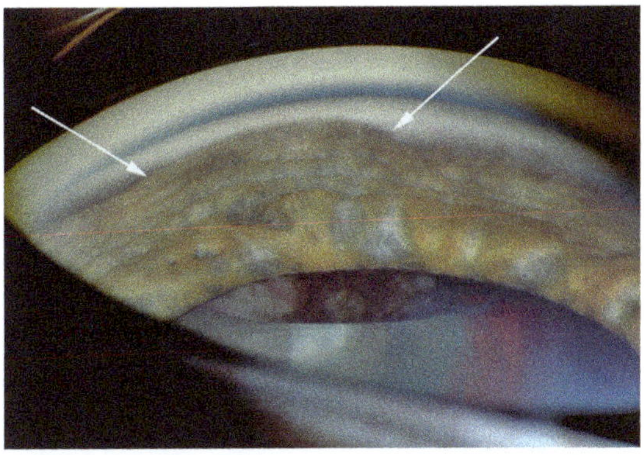

Fig. 7.27 Peripheral anterior synechiae due to a tumor of the ciliary body (*between the arrows*) pushing the iris forward

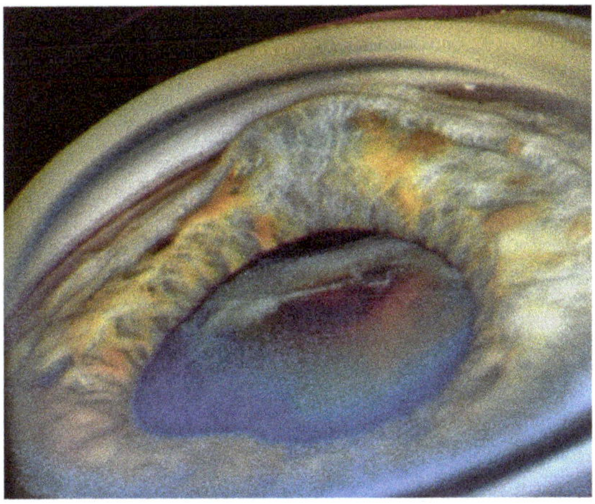

Fig. 7.28 Tumor of the ciliary body pushing the peripheral iris into the chamber angle. Note the heavily pigmented trabecular meshwork

In eyes with endothelial posterior polymorphous dystrophy of the cornea (Schlichting).

7.2.1.3 Without Pupillary Block, but with an Anterior Pushing Mechanism

In eyes with aqueous misdirection, "malignant" reaction. The misdirection of the aqueous humor into the posterior compartments (behind the lens, into the vitreous body) of the eye pushes the lens-iris-diaphragm anteriorly. Uveal effusion is an additional component.

In eyes with iris or ciliary body cysts or tumors (Figs. 7.27, 7.28, and 7.29). Their real extent and size are preferentially visualized by

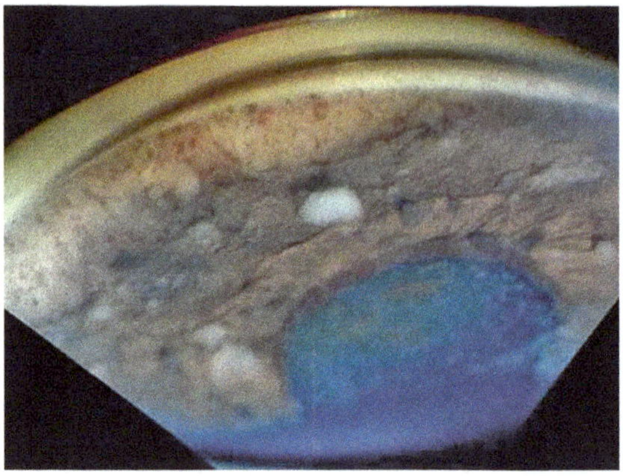

Fig. 7.29 Masses of tumor tissue occluding at least the inferior half of the chamber angle (tapioca melanoma)

UBM. Multiple, enlarging cysts may lead to a pseudoplateau iris syndrome. In contrast to a plateau iris syndrome, the peripheral iris is more bumpy, the closure is localized to only a few clock hours, and there is usually more pigment in the visible trabecular meshwork. Treatment is also different: the aim is to rupture the cysts or to remove them surgically. Tumors require individual treatment.

In eyes with silicone oil or expanding air/gas mixture (Fig. 7.30) after vitrectomy.

Because it is so important: P. Palmberg listed the reasons for missing the diagnosis angle-closure disease:

1. Not performing gonioscopy at all when angle closure is not suspected
2. Not performing gonioscopy in a dark room with care to avoid letting the slit lamp beam enter the pupil
3. Performing gonioscopy with a Goldmann-style lens (large diameter), which, by creating suction on the cornea, increases the IOP and opens closed angles
4. Inadvertently pressing on the cornea with a Zeiss-style goniolens (indentation lens) inducing corneal folds
5. Misinterpreting the pigment of Sampaolesi's line as the pigmented trabecular meshwork in an angle that is in reality closed

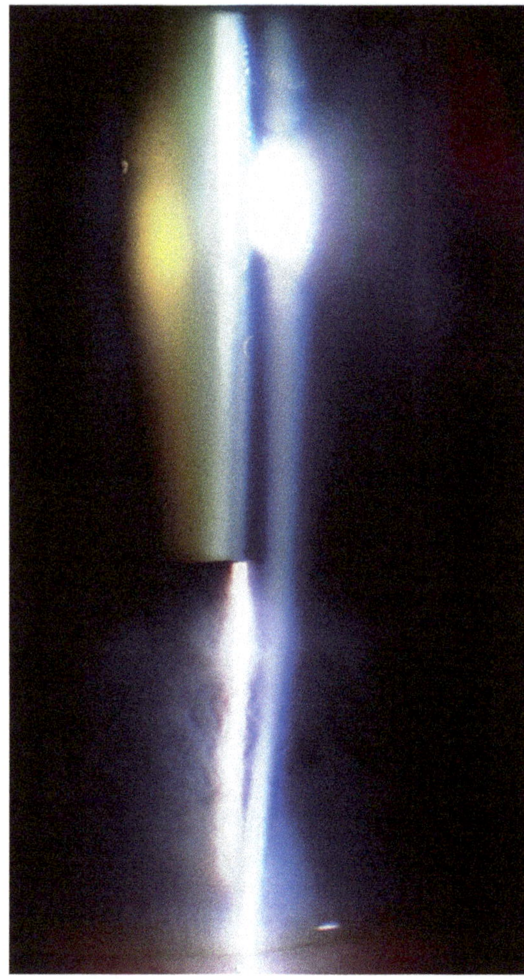

Fig. 7.30 Slitlamp photograph of an eye filled with sulfur hexafluoride gas after vitrectomy showing a very shallow central and peripheral anterior chamber. Depending on the gas used check the IOP in those eyes regularly!

Bibliography

Alward WL, Longmuir RA (2008) Color atlas of gonioscopy, 2nd edn. American Academy of Ophthalmology, San Francisco

Debrouwere V, Stalmans P, van Calster J, Spileers W, Zeyen T, Stalmans I (2012) Outcomes of different management options for malignant glaucoma: a retrospective review. Graefes Arch Clin Exp Ophthalmol 250:131–141

Dorairaj S, Tello C, Liebman JM, Ritch R (2007) Narrow angles and angle closure: anatomic reasons for earlier closure of the superior portion of the iridocorneal angle. Arch Ophthalmol 125:734–739

European Glaucoma Society (2008) Terminology and guidelines for glaucoma, 3rd edn. European Glaucoma Society/Dogma, Savona

Fang A, Yang X, Nie L, Qu J (2010) Endoscopically controlled goniosynechialysis in managing synechial angle-closure glaucoma. J Glaucoma 19:19–23

Foster PJ, Buhrmann R, Quigley HA, Johnson GJ (2002) The definition and classification of glaucoma in prevalence surveys. Br J Ophthalmol 86:238–242

Foster PJ, Aung T, Nolan WP, Machin D, Baasanhu J, Khaw PT, Alsbirk PH, Lee PS, Seah SKL, Johnson GJ (2004) Defining "occludable" angles in population surveys: drainage angle width, peripheral anterior synechiae, and glaucomatous optic neuropathy in East Asian people. Br J Ophthalmol 88:486–490

Mansouri K, Burgener ND, Bagnoud M, Shaarawy T (2009) A prospective ultrasound biomicroscopy evaluation of changes in anterior segment morphology following laser iridotomy in European eyes. Eye (Lond) 23:2046–2051

Nongpiur ME, Ku JY, Aung T (2011) Angle closure glaucoma: a mechanistic review. Curr Opin Ophthalmol 22:96–101

Palmberg P (2007) Shedding light on gonioscopy. Arch Ophthalmol 125:1417–1418

Quigley HA (2009a) What's the choroid got to do with angle closure (editorial). Arch Ophthalmol 127:693–694

Quigley HA (2009b) Angle-closure glaucoma – simpler answers to complex mechanisms: LXVI Edward Jackson Memorial Lecture. Am J Ophthalmol 148:657–669

Quigley HA (2010) The iris is a sponge: a cause of angle closure. Ophthalmology 117:1–2

Quigley HA (2011) Glaucoma. Lancet 377:1367–1377

Quigley HA, Silver DM, Friedman DS et al (2009) Iris cross-sectional area decreases with pupil dilation and its dynamic behaviour is a risk factor in angle closure. J Glaucoma 18:173–179

Ravi T, Walland MJ, Parikh RS (2011) Clear lens extraction in angle closure glaucoma. Curr Opin Ophthalmol 22: 110–114

Sharma T, Low S, Foster PJ (2009) The classification of primary angle-closure glaucoma. In: Krieglstein GK, Weinreb RN (eds) Essentials in ophthalmology, glaucoma. Springer, Berlin, pp 41–49

Shukla S, Damji KF, Harasymowycz P, Chialant D, Kent JS, Chevrier R, Buhrmann R, Marshall D, Pan Y, Hodge W (2008) Clinical features distinguishing angle closure from pseudoplateau versus plateau iris. Br J Ophthalmol 92:340–344

Wang BS, Narayanaswamy A, Amerasinghe N, Zheng C, He M, Chan YH, Nongpiur ME, Friedman DS, Aung T (2011) Increased iris thickness and association with primary angle closure glaucoma. Br J Ophthalmol 95: 46–50

Weinreb RN, Friedman DS (2006) Angle closure and angle closure glaucoma: reports and consensus statements of the 3rd Global AIGS Consensus Meeting on angle closure glaucoma. Kugler, The Hague

8 Additional Examinations to Gonioscopy

The systems described below are used for examination of the chamber angle and the anterior segment of the eye. They provide cross-sectional images and allow objective quantitative assessment. Do they support us with additional information to gonioscopy? When are these devices recommended? What are their limitations?

8.1 AS-OCT

AS-OCT stands for "anterior segment optical coherence tomography." It is a noninvasive, noncontact method for examining different parts of the eye. AS-OCT was developed for the anterior segment and was first described by Izatt et al. in 1994. The principle of the method is similar to that of ultrasonography, except using light instead of sound, which is emitted and reflected. In contrast to retinal OCT, anterior segment OCT uses higher power and a longer wavelength (1,310 nm) allowing greater penetration. Scanning through an opaque cornea is possible.

The patient is in a sitting position during examination of several cross sections. Angle grading, and peripheral and central iris configuration are easily demonstrated. Several biometric parameters can be calculated automatically by the image processing software: central anterior chamber depth (ACD), anterior chamber volume (ACV), iridolenticular contact area, iris volume-to-length ratio, angle recess (angle recess area, ARA), the interspur distance, the angle opening distance at 250, 500 or 750 μm (AOD) and the trabecular-iris spur area at 500 μm (TISA 500).

The resolution differs between the systems, but it is axial in the range 18–25 μm and transverse in the range 20–100 μm. The trabecular meshwork per se cannot be visualized; therefore the scleral spur is the landmark in the majority of the cases.

HD-OCT (high definition) offers a higher resolution and a better definition of the angle structures, but has a limited field of view.

One major advantage is that the examination is even possible under very low light conditions so that the pupil size is unaffected. Qualitative assessment of the angle during bright light and dark may be shown dynamically.

Since coherent light is absorbed by the heavily pigmented posterior layer of the iris the imaging of AS-OCT is limited to tissue anterior to this layer.

The big disadvantage is that only one single meridian is examined, in contrast to dynamic gonioscopy, where the complete 360° are assessed. Remember: only in eyes with >270° of nonvisibility

C. Faschinger, A. Hommer, *Gonioscopy*,
DOI 10.1007/978-3-642-28610-0_8, © Springer-Verlag Berlin Heidelberg 2012

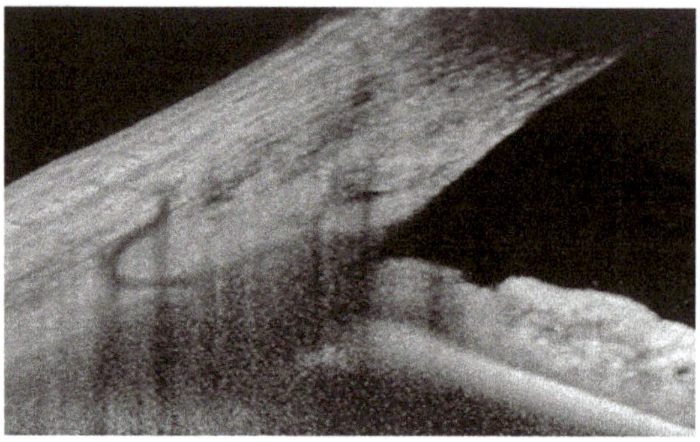

Fig. 8.1 AS-OCT of a regular chamber angle. Schlemm's canal and a transscleral collector channel are visible

of the trabecular meshwork can you diagnose angle-closure suspect! (Figs. 8.1 and 8.2).

8.2 UBM

Ultrasound biomicroscopy (UBM) is a noninvasive contact method that uses ultrasound for the examination of the chamber angle. It was first described by Palvin et al. in 1992. The transducer emits short acoustic pulses that generate echoes. These are reflected by ocular tissues, translated into voltages and converted into pixel intensity for to generate the cross-sectional images. The high frequencies (in the range 35–50 MHz) emitted by the ultrasound probe's transducer provide a high resolution of up to 25 μm axially and 50 μm transversally. UBM has a greater depth of penetration than AS-OCT, because acoustic waves are not blocked by the pigmented iris epithelium. The depth of penetration is about 5 mm allowing examination of the ciliary body, ciliary sulcus and other structures posterior to the iris, e.g., iris cysts or ciliary body melanoma. The scleral spur is the only constant landmark (Figs. 8.3 and 8.4).

A disadvantage is the fact that the examinations have to be performed in a supine position with a liquid-filled cup (water) or a single-use water-filled balloon probe cover. The cup can distort the angle configuration. Parameters such as ACD, trabecular–iris angle, AOD at 250 or 500 μm from the scleral spur (AOD 250 or AOD 500), iris thickness, and ARA can be calculated.

There is high agreement between gonioscopy and UBM in detecting iridotrabecular appositions.

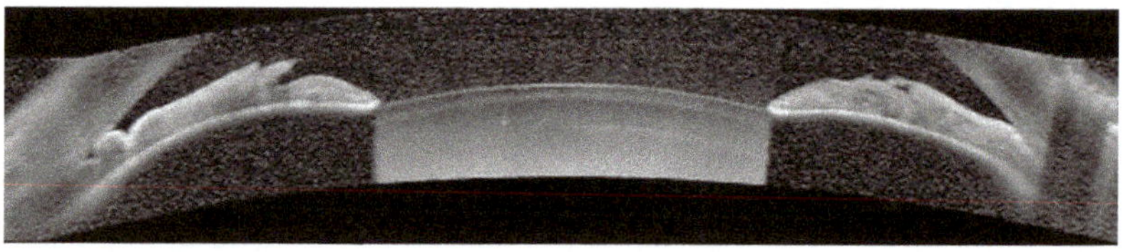

Fig. 8.2 AS-OCT of a closed chamber angle (180° cut). The temporal part shows a thick peripheral iris roll (Fuchs) closing the angle. Nasally the iris closes the angle completely

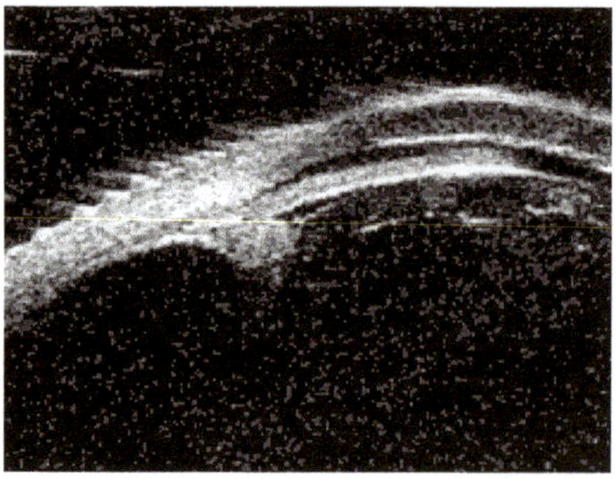

Fig. 8.3 UBM of the right eye of a patient with acute angle closure attack. The iris is very close to the corneal endothelium, and the chamber angle is closed

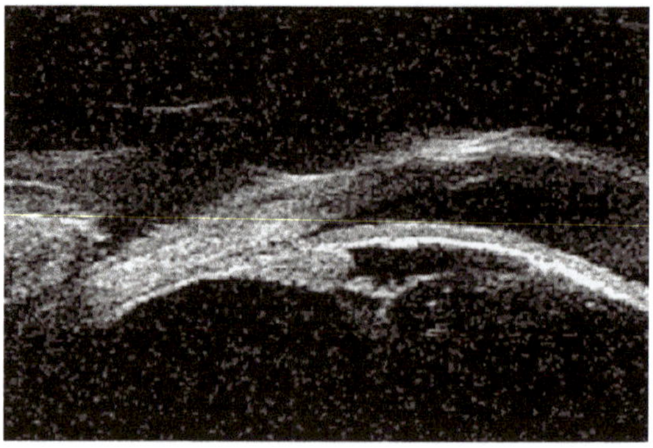

Fig. 8.4 UBM of the left eye of the same patient. The chamber is deeper than in the right eye, but there are also peripheral anterior synechiae

Again, it is an advantage to perform the examinations in very low light conditions (UBM dark room provocation test). UBM even works in premature infants, so that differences from angles in adults can be studied. One of its most useful applications is in differentiating the causes of angle closure and it is also useful in congenital glaucoma with developmental disorders or diseases with hazy corneas. Dynamic/indentation gonioscopy can even be performed during UBM by applying mild pressure on the peripheral cornea with the skirt of the eyecup.

8.3 Pentacam-Scheimpflug

This system uses a rotating Scheimpflug camera that takes up to 50 slit images of the anterior segment of the eye in less than 2 s. A second camera corrects artifacts resulting from eye movements. Besides corneal and lens data (depending on the size of the pupil), the ACD and the ACV are calculated (Fig. 8.5). An ACV value of less than 113 mm^3 indicates an increased risk. Using this as the cut-off value provides a 90% sensitivity and 88% specificity for detecting narrow angles.

Based on the thickness values of the cornea, corrected IOP values are generated. Direct visualization of the chamber angle is not possible. However, the configuration of the iris (flat, forward bowing, concave) and the distance from the iris margin to the anterior lens surface are demonstrated well. New software compares the actual values of the chamber angularity, depth and volume to values in a standard database.

8.4 Orbscan

The anterior segment is scanned by a slit-beam system comparable to a Scheimpflug slit lamp scanning system. Forty images are produced by a calibrated video camera with up to 240 data points per slit of all surfaces (cornea, iris, lens). The maximal resolution is up to 2 μm in the central zone. Corneal thickness, ACD and ACV are calculated. The chamber angle per se is not quantified, but an estimation of the chamber angle is possible.

8.5 EyeCam

All the devices mentioned above produce cross-sectional views of one point through the angle. The EyeCam provides 90° of angle visualization per image, but no quantitative analyses. The pictures are in color easing the detection of the landmarks of the angle. The EyeCam is a modification of the RetCam. The camera provides a view quite similar to direct gonioscopy with the Koeppe lens.

In summary, the examinations with these systems provide help in understanding several specific anatomical, pathophysiological and functional conditions. Grading of the angle width by means of gonioscopy is subjective. Image devices

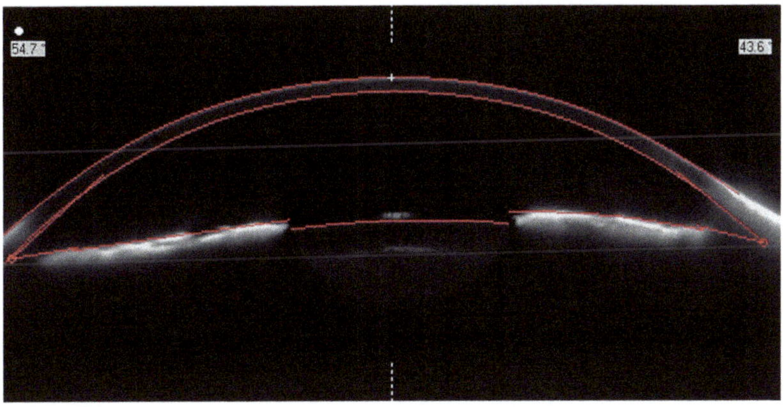

Fig. 8.5 Result of a Scheimpflug camera examination in a myopic eye (–5 diopters) with a gonioscopically wide open chamber angle: temporal angle 54.7°, nasal angle 43.6°, anterior chamber depth 4.26 mm, anterior chamber volume 269 mm^3

provide objective data with low variability and high reproducibility. Only AS-OCT and UBM visualize the chamber angle per se including anatomical details. For pathological changes behind the iris, the UBM is very helpful.

Some of the devices are possibly useful in screening, especially for primary angle closure. AS-OCT and UBM are invaluable tools for differentiating cysts from solid tumors of the anterior segment. None of them replaces gonioscopy. It is not their aim, but they may give important additional insight.

Bibliography

Auffarth GU, Tetz MR, Biazid Y, Völcker HE (1997) Measuring anterior chamber depth with the Orbscan Topography System. J Cataract Refract Surg 23: 1351–1355

Console JW, Sakata LM, Aung T, Friedman DS, He M (2008) Quantitative analysis of anterior segment optical coherence tomography images: the Zhongshan angle assessment program. Br J Ophthalmol 92:1612–1616

Dada T, Gadia R, Sharma A, Ichhpujani P, Bail SJ, Bhartija S, Panda A (2011) Ultrasound biomicroscopy in glaucoma. Surv Ophthalmol 56:433–450

Foster PJ, Buhrmann R, Quigley HA, Johnson GJ (2002) The definition and classification of glaucoma in prevalence surveys. Br J Ophthalmol 86:238–242

Grewal DS, Brar GS, Jain R, Grewal SP (2011) Comparison of Scheimpflug imaging and spectral domain anterior segment optical coherence tomography for detection of narrow anterior chamber angles. Eye 25:603–611

Izatt JA, Hee MR, Swanson EA, Lin CP, Huang D, Schuman JS, Puliafito CA, Fujimoto JG (1994) Micrometer-scale resolution imaging of the anterior eye in vivo with optical coherence tomography. Arch Ophthalmol 112:1584–1589

Kobayashi H, Kiryu J, Kobayashi K, Kondo T (1997) Ultrasound biomicroscopic measurements of anterior chamber angle in premature infants. Br J Ophthalmol 81:460–464

Konstantinopoulos A, Hossain P, Anderson DF (2007) Recent advances in ophthalmic anterior segment imaging: a new era for ophthalmic diagnosis? Br J Ophthalmol 91:551–557

Palvin CJ, Harasiewicz K, Sherar MD, Foster FS (1991) Clinical use of ultrasound biomicroscopy. Ophthalmology 98:287–295

Palvin CJ, Harasiewicz K, Foster FS (1992) Ultrasound biomicroscopy of anterior segment structures in normal and glaucomatous eyes. Am J Ophthalmol 113:381–389

Perera SA, Quek DT, Baskaran M, Tun TA, Kumar RS, Friedman DS, Aung T (2010) Demonstration of angle widening using EyeCam after laser peripheral iridotomy in eyes with angle closure. Am J Ophthalmol 149:903–907

Quigley HA (2010) The iris is a sponge: a cause of angle closure. Ophthalmology 117:1–2

Reisdorf S (2011) Scheimpflugkamera – Messprinzip und Anwendungsmöglichkeiten. Z Prakt Augenheilkd 32: 557–565

9 Laser Treatments in the Chamber Angle

LASER is an acronym that stands for *l*ight *a*mplification of *s*timulated *e*mission of *r*adiation. In simple terms it is parallel light of a certain wavelength. Laser light is used in different wavelengths to treat glaucoma. Tissues that can be treated are the iris, the trabecular meshwork to improve outflow facility and the ciliary body processes to reduce aqueous humor production.

9.1 Thermal Lasers

9.1.1 Laser Trabeculoplasty

In laser trabeculoplasty with thermal lasers, which include the argon laser in continuous wave mode (wavelength 488–514 nm; argon laser trabeculoplasty) and the diode laser (wavelength 810 nm; diode laser trabeculoplasty), heat from the laser beam induces burns, causing inflammation, which later forms scars. The trabecular tissue between two scarring spots is therefore open and outflow increases (mechanical theory).

The spots have a size of 50 μm. The duration of each pulse is 0.1 s. Spots (50–100, original count by Wise and Witter) are placed between the nonfunctional (anterior) and the functional (posterior) trabecular meshwork around 360°. The duration time depends on the amount of pigment and is between 400 and 1,200 mW. The laser spots should induce a grayish color in the trabecular meshwork, and tiny gas bubbles are possible. Application too close or at the ciliary band should be avoided. Peripheral anterior synechiae at a regular distance are an unmistakable sign of an improperly applied argon laser trabeculoplasty. Use a contact lens which is designed for trabeculoplasty (Fig. 9.1).

9.1.2 Argon Laser Suturolysis

If the (non-resorbable) sutures of the scleral flap in filtration surgery are too tight almost no filtering bleb will develop. Sometimes a gentle massage will help for a short time. It is advisable to perform a lysis of the black 10-0 nylon suture using a laser. Anesthetize the eye, and hold a Hoskins lens on the conjunctiva directly upon the suture to get a larger view. A diameter of 50 μm and a duration of 0.1–0.15 s are good settings. Never open more than one suture a day and check the outflow immediately. A filtering bleb should arise. At least one suture has to remain (Figs. 9.2 and 9.3).

9.1.3 Argon Laser Peripheral Iridoplasty

Argon laser peripheral iridoplasty is a method to flatten the steep iris in plateau-iris configuration or plateau-iris syndrome. The heat of the laser burns the iris tissue which then shrinks, and this contraction opens the angle, thus avoiding iridotrabecular contact or formation of synechiae. The angle widens immediately. Due to the nerve supply to the iris this procedure might be painful, so inform the patient in advance. If necessary use a peribulbar block. The settings are: 0.5 ms, 500 μm diameter and about five

C. Faschinger, A. Hommer, *Gonioscopy*,
DOI 10.1007/978-3-642-28610-0_9, © Springer-Verlag Berlin Heidelberg 2012

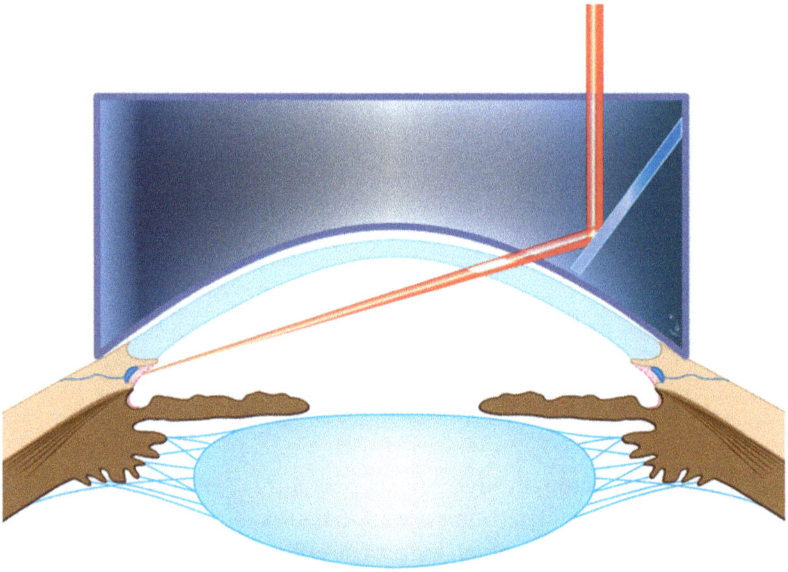

Fig. 9.1 A contact lens designed for trabeculoplasty is placed on the cornea and the laser beam is exactly focused between the non-functional and the functional trabecular meshwork

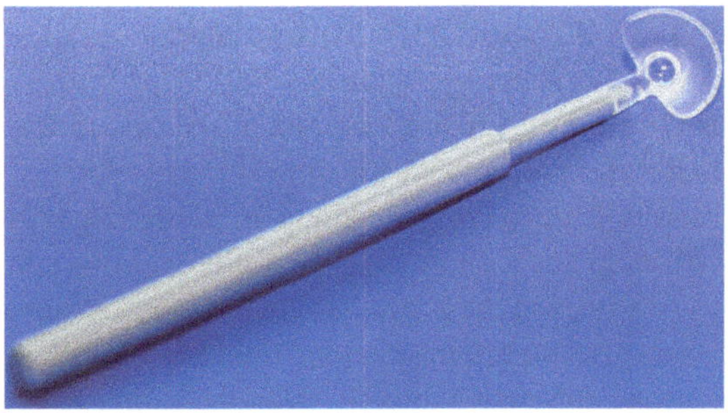

Fig. 9.2 Hoskins lens for suturolysis. The suture is enlarged and can be clear visualized

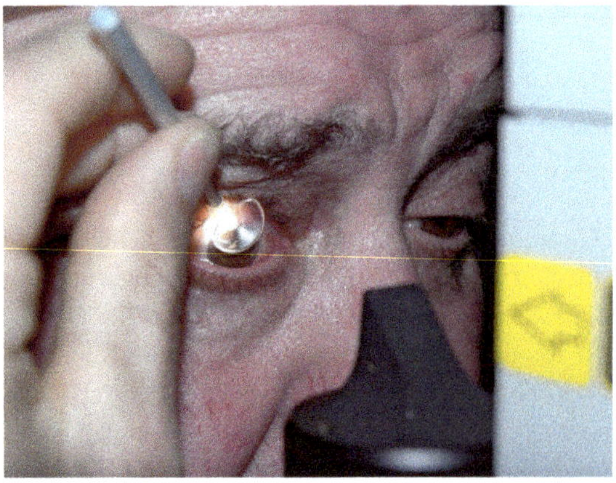

Fig. 9.3 Argon laser suturolysis. Using the Hoskins lens one suture is easily opened and a filtering bleb should arise immediately

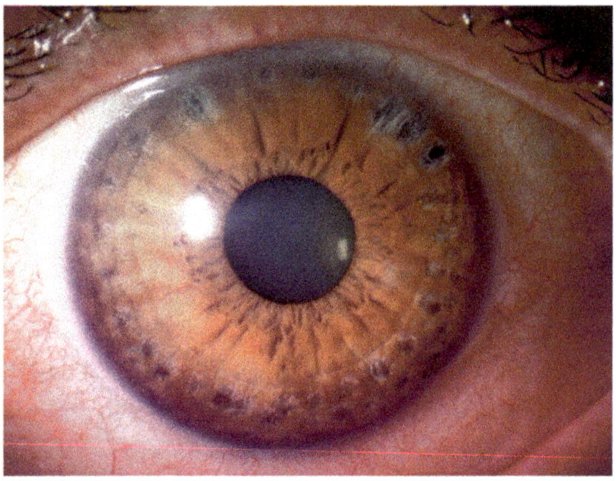

Fig. 9.4 There are two patent Nd:YAG iridotomies (11 and 2 o'clock) and several scars in the periphery of the iris after argon laser peripheral iridoplasty in two rows. Before the iridoplasty the IOP increased despite patent iridotomies when the pupil was dilated

to seven spots per quadrant. Try to apply the spots as peripherally as possible. Sometimes you will need two lines to flatten the iris appropriately. Sometimes a wider pupil than before may result (Fig. 9.4).

9.1.4 Transscleral Cyclophotocoagulation

A diode laser (wavelength 810 nm) is applied transsclerally to destroy parts of the ciliary processes to decrease the production of aqueous humor. The probe automatically gives you the appropriate distance to the limbus. The treatment involves the application of 20–25 spots with 2,000 mW power and 2,000 ms exposure time over three-quarters of the circumference. Spare the 3 and 9 o'clock positions because of the long anterior ciliary vessels (Fig. 9.5). If you hear a "pop" (a sign of microexplosion of tissue) the energy level is too high. Better efficacy and safety may be reached with a controlled application of the laser spots (*co*ntrolled *co*agulation, COCO; power 5,000 mW, exposure time 500 ms).

9.1.5 Endoscopic Cyclophotocoagulation, Endocycloplasty

A 20-gauge curved laser probe (diode, 810 nm, with a fiber optic camera) is inserted into the eye posterior to the iris to treat the ciliary processes. It is primarily used in combination with phacoemulsification. The ciliary processes are partially destroyed by the heat and will produce less aqueous humor. Each ciliary processus is treated over at least 270°.

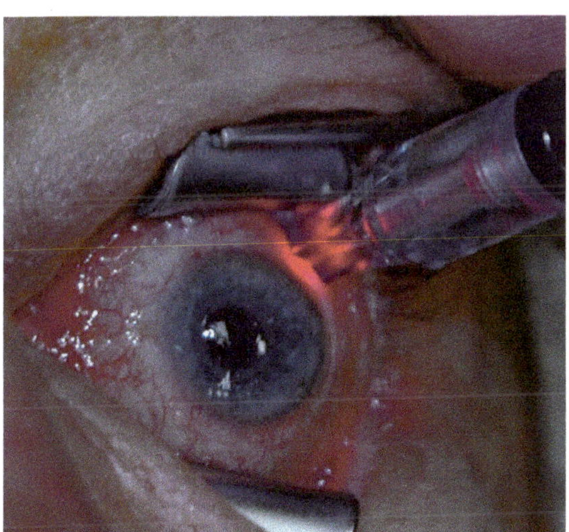

Fig. 9.5 The probe of the diode laser is set perpendicular on the limbal region. The laser acts 1.5 mm behind. The red light is from the aiming beam

Endocycloplasty is the same procedure, but with less power (250–350 mW), so no destruction but only shrinkage of the ciliary processes will occur. Indications are eyes with cataract and plateau-iris syndrome.

9.2 Non-thermal Lasers

9.2.1 Selective Laser Trabeculoplasty

In selective laser trabeculoplasty a frequency-doubled Nd:YAG laser (wavelength 532 nm) in pulsed mode is used and the target of treatment are the melanocytes of the trabecular meshwork. The treatment leads to the release of cytokines, activation of macrophages and disassembly of the intercellular junctions. The destructive elements are much less than in argon laser trabeculoplasty. Different settings for the laser beam parameters are used. Because of the larger diameter, exact focusing is not as important as in argon laser trabeculoplasty. The center of the large beam should be aimed at the trabecular meshwork (Fig. 9.6). Do not cover the iris. The delivered energy is 100-fold less than in argon laser trabeculoplasty. The exposure time is preset and is 3 ns. In a heavily pigmented trabeculum you will need less energy, and a treatment over 90° might be sufficient. The therapy end-points are

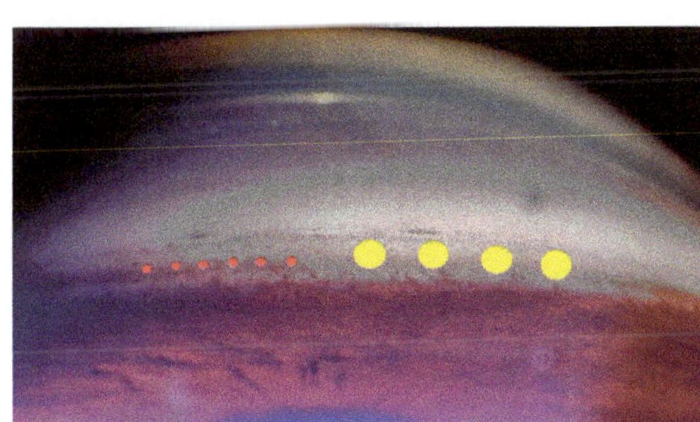

Fig. 9.6 The argon laser spots in argon laser trabeculoplasty are located between the functional and non-functional trabecular meshwork (*red dots*) and the Nd:YAG laser spots in selective laser trabeculoplasty are located on the functional and non-functional trabecular meshwork (*yellow dots*)

Table 9.1 The numbers of spots, power, spot sizes and exposure times for argon laser trabeculoplasty and selective laser trabeculoplasty, their ratios (Fig. 9.5)

	Argon laser trabeculoplasty	Selective laser trabeculoplasty	Ratio
Number of spots	50 (180°)–100 (360°)	50 (180°)–100 (360°)	1:1
Energy	400–1,200 mW	0.3–2.0 mJ	1:100
Spot size	50 μm	400 μm (preset)	1:8
Exposition time	100,000,000 ns (0.1 s)	3 ns (preset)	1:33,000,000

cavitation bubbles ("champagne bubbles"), then the energy is scaled down by 0.1 mJ. A probable benefit is its effectiveness when repeated, even several times.

In laser trabeculoplasty, no matter if thermal or non-thermal, you have to use contact lenses designed for trabeculoplasty. They should have no magnification factor, because this could alter the beam diameter and energy (over- or under-treatment). Always titrate the energy level in accordance with angle pigmentation in the different quadrants. An important condition is an open angle with a visible trabecular meshwork! A recent report by the American Academy of Ophthalmology revealed no superiority of any particular form of laser trabeculoplasty.

The laser settings for argon laser trabeculoplasty and selective laser trabeculoplasty are compared in Table 9.1.

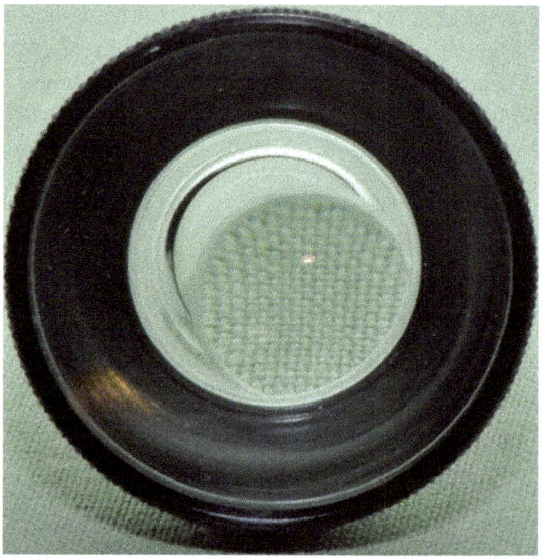

Fig. 9.7 For laser peripheral iridotomy use a lens designed for the procedure. Most of these lenses have a thicker part which enlarges the view of the iris tissue

9.3 Disruptive Lasers

The Nd:YAG laser with a wavelength of 1,064 nm disrupts tissues, e.g. the posterior lens capsule or the iris. The surgical removal of iris tissue to create a hole is called iridectomy; the creation of a hole using a laser is called iridotomy. An iridectomy, first described by Graefe in 1857, or an iridotomy heals an eye with a pupillary block.

Use a contact lens that is designed for iridotomy (laser peripheral iridotomy; Fig. 9.7). Search for a crypt between two trabecular tissue structures at the base of the iris where the stromal layer of the iris is thin. Then apply a few shots on the iris until aqueous humor and pigment blow out of the hole. One patent hole of 200 μm is enough. At what position? Try to avoid the 10 and 2 o'clock positions. Refractive phenomena of the tear film at the lid margin may induce stray light or the patient may complain of a positive dysphotopsia in the form of a dark crescent in the inferior part of the visual field. At 12 o'clock gas bubbles may obscure the view.

A thick iris (brown eyes) might be flattened and thinned by pretreatment with an argon laser. The burns will shrink the tissue (Fig. 9.8)

In eyes which have undergone a deep sclerectomy, a "goniopuncture" of Descemet's window might be necessary to enhance the outflow into the scleral lake.

9.4 Excimer Lasers

Excimer lasers (wavelength range 193–308 nm) ablate tissue with almost no thermal side effects. After filling of the anterior chamber with an

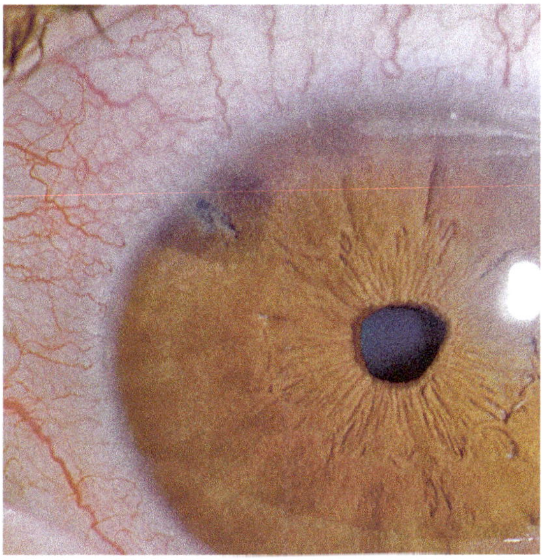

Fig. 9.8 Pretreatment of a thick brown iris with the argon laser to flatten and shrink the tissue. The Nd:YAG laser is then used to create a hole

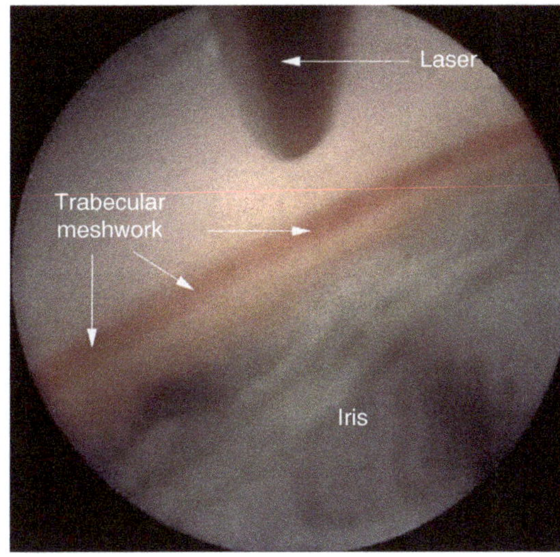

Fig. 9.10 The endoscopic probe is inside the anterior chamber. The chamber angle is wide open with a relatively strong pigmented trabecular meshwork and a broad anterior ciliary band (Courtesy J. Funk)

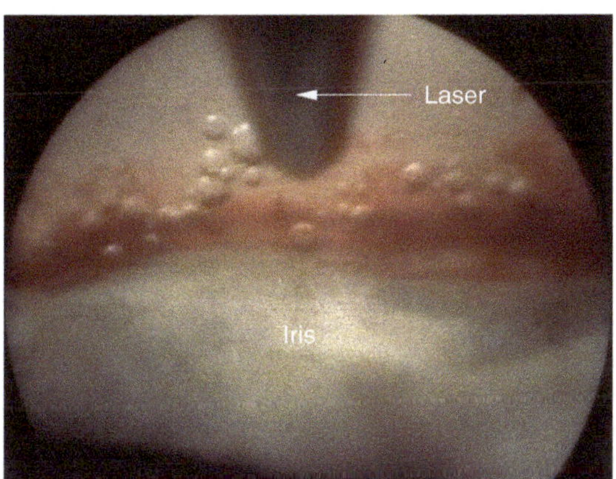

Fig. 9.9 Air bubbles and blood are typical signs immediately after the laser application (Courtesy J. Funk)

ophthalmic viscoelastic device, a laser probe (endoscopically guided) is brought into the eye. The trabecular meshwork is ablated from the inside and opened up to Schlemm's canal by a few spots (spot size 200 μm, ten spots within 90°) (excimer laser trabeculotomy, ab interno; Figs. 9.9 and 9.10). An important condition is a wide open angle, so combination with a phacoemulsification of the lens is advisable.

Bibliography

Alward WL, Longmuir RA (2008) Color atlas of gonioscopy, 2nd edn. American Academy of Ophthalmology, San Francisco

European Glaucoma Society (2008) Terminology and guidelines for glaucoma, 3rd edn. European Glaucoma Society/Dogma, Savona

Latina MA, Tumbocon JA (2001) Selective laser trabeculoplasty: a new treatment option for open angle glaucoma. Curr Opin Ophthalmol 13:94–96

Samples JR, Singh K, Lin SH et al (2011) Laser trabeculoplasty for open-angle glaucoma. A report by the American Academy of Ophthalmology. Ophthalmology 118:2296–2302

Wilmsmeyer S, Philippin H, Funk J (2006) Excimer laser trabeculotomy: a new, minimally invasive procedure for patients with glaucoma. Graefes Arch Clin Exp Ophthalmol 244:670–676

Wise BJ, Witter SL (1979) Argon laser therapy for open-angle glaucoma. Arch Ophthalmol 97:319–322

Surgery in the Chamber Angle 10

Many surgical procedures in glaucoma have the aim of improving outflow facility by different means. Only a few aim to reduce the production of aqueous humor. Some of them are more, some less and some minimally invasive.

Is gonioscopy of informational value before, during and/or after an operation? Definitely, yes! You need to know about the anatomical status. Some of these procedures require an open chamber angle, and therefore they are preferably performed in combination with phacoemulsification of the lens.

10.1 Filtration or Penetrating Surgery (Trabeculectomy)

After preparation of the conjunctiva, Tenon's capsule and the scleral flap, a tiny full-thickness part of the cornea, the trabecular meshwork and sclera is excised to create a bypass flow below the Tenon–conjunctiva complex, called a filtering bleb (Fig. 10.1). It is highly advisable to perform a peripheral iridectomy to avoid blockage of the new fistula.

If the IOP is the same postoperatively as it was preoperatively, the anterior chamber is the same depth, there is no filtering bleb and the pupil is possibly slightly distorted to the site of the scleral flap, a gonioscopy should be done. One might find the iris trapped in the fistula, and no further outflow is possible (Figs. 10.2 and 10.3). Revision is mandatory.

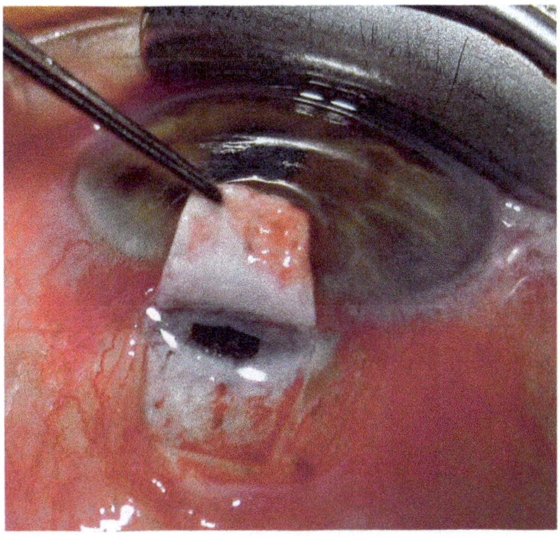

Fig. 10.1 Opening of the scleral flap shows the hole after excision of a tiny part of the sclera, cornea and the trabecular meshwork. To prevent occlusion of this hole by the iris a peripheral iridectomy has been performed, so the ciliary processes are visible

If the bleb is well functioning, the chamber angle shows a rectangular excision with a flat and tiny slit between the sclera and the flap (Fig. 10.4).

10.2 Non-penetrating Surgery

10.2.1 Deep Sclerectomy

After preparation of the conjunctiva, Tenon's capsule and the scleral flap, a second, deep and a little bit smaller scleral flap is created and excised.

C. Faschinger, A. Hommer, *Gonioscopy*,
DOI 10.1007/978-3-642-28610-0_10,

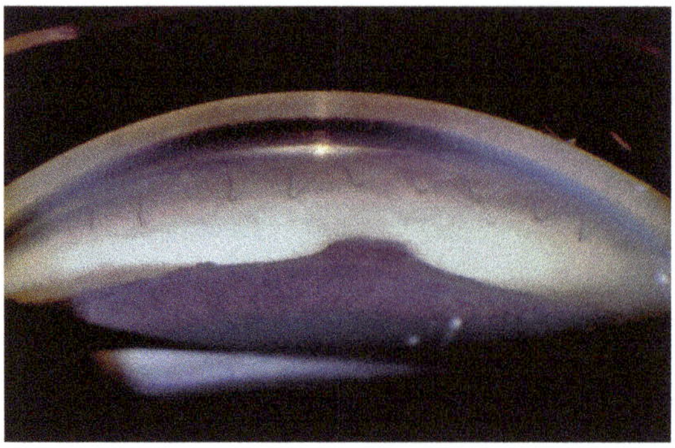

Fig. 10.2 The iris is trapped in the excision site of the trabeculectomy. The running nylon suture of the conjunctiva/Tenon's capsule at the limbus is visible. Revision is mandatory because outflow through the fistula is blocked. The patient had experienced a blunt trauma

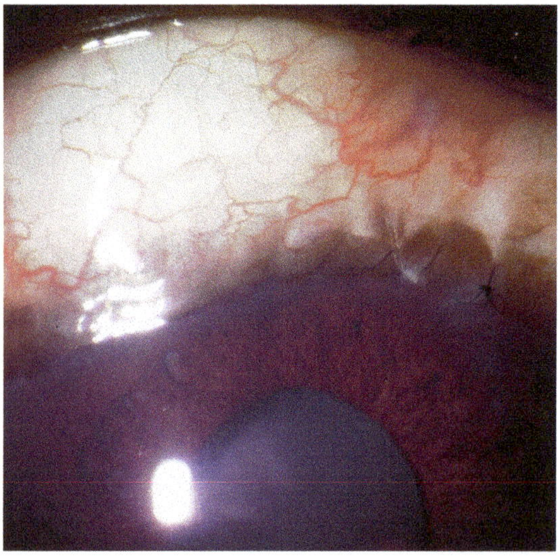

Fig. 10.3 Filtering bleb with running nylon suture at the limbus in the same eye as shown in Fig. 10.2. Note the slight distortion of the pupil towards the site of filtration because of trapping of the peripheral iris

The preparation proceeds into the corneal tissue performing a "Descemet's window," a clear rectangular area where aqueous humor should "percolate" from the anterior chamber into the newly created reservoir between the sclera ("scleral lake") and the conjunctiva, producing a filtering bleb (Fig. 10.5). In gonioscopy, Descemet's window can be seen clearly. On gentle pressure with the contact lens Descemet's membrane and the endothelium will wave lake a sail in the wind.

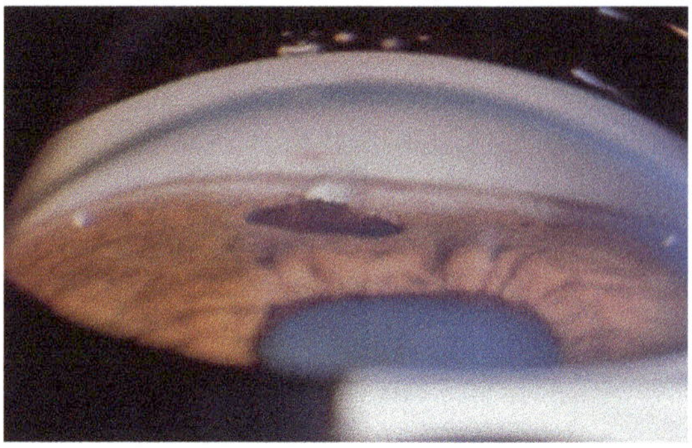

Fig. 10.4 Excision site after trabeculectomy in the chamber angle including a part of the scleral spur and the posterior, pigmented trabecular meshwork. The bright white sclera of the inner wall of the scleral flap is visible

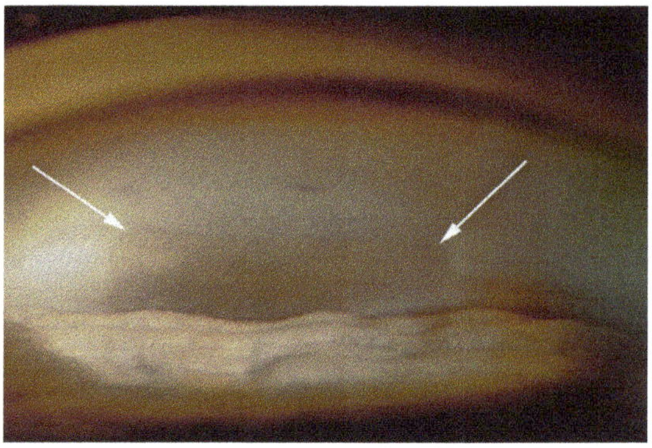

Fig. 10.5 Rectangular Descemet's window (edges are marked by *arrows*) after resection of a deep scleral flap (Courtesy A. Mermoud)

10.2.2 Viscocanalostomy

The first steps are the same as in deep sclerectomy. After excision of the deep scleral flap, the ostia of Schlemm's canal are widened with a viscoelastic agent (an ophthalmic viscosurgical device, OVD), doubling their diameter. Watertight closure of the scleral flap avoids a filtering bleb. Gonioscopy reveals the same as in deep sclerectomy.

10.2.3 Viscotrabeculotomy

As in viscocanalostomy, the ostia of Schlemm's canal are widened, but afterwards specific cannulas are introduced into the canal and injection of the OVD will cause some parts of the trabecular meshwork to rupture. The scleral flap is closed very tightly so that no filtering bleb will develop.

10.3 Implants

10.3.1 Canaloplasty

The preparation is the same as that for visco-canalostomy, but the entire Schlemm's canal is cannulated with a small, flexible fiber optic microcatheter. A non-resorbable suture is connected to the fiber, the fiber is pulled back and the suture is knotted under tension. The septae of Schlemm's canal are disrupted and the canal is opened because of the tension of the suture. In gonioscopy the blue suture might be detected in the posterior trabecular meshwork.

10.3.2 iStent Trabecular Micro-Bypass

A small, L-shaped stent (1 × 0.5 × 0.25 mm, snorkel opening 120 μm) made of titanium is implanted ab interno in the trabecular meshwork and Schlemm's canal (Fig. 10.6). It is easily detectable by gonioscopy.

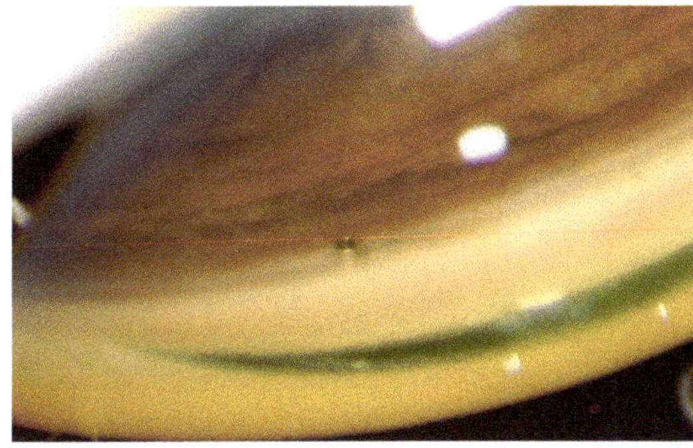

Fig. 10.6 iStent positioned exactly in the chamber angle at the functional trabecular meshwork (Courtesy S. Windsor, Glaucos)

10.3.3 Ex-PRESS Mini Glaucoma Shunt

A 3-mm long tube with an external diameter of 400 μm (27 gauge) and a lumen of 50 μm is implanted at the site where the tissue would be excised in trabeculectomy. A spur on the surface of the tube avoids extrusion and a plate intrusion. An iridectomy is not necessary.

10.3.4 SOLX Gold Shunt

A 24-carat gold plate (3.2 mm wide posteriorly and 2.4 mm wide anteriorly, 5.2 mm long) with many tiny perforations and microchannels is implanted in the supraciliary/suprachoroidal space to enhance the outflow. Newer devices (GMS Plus) with increased thickness and more pores are offered.

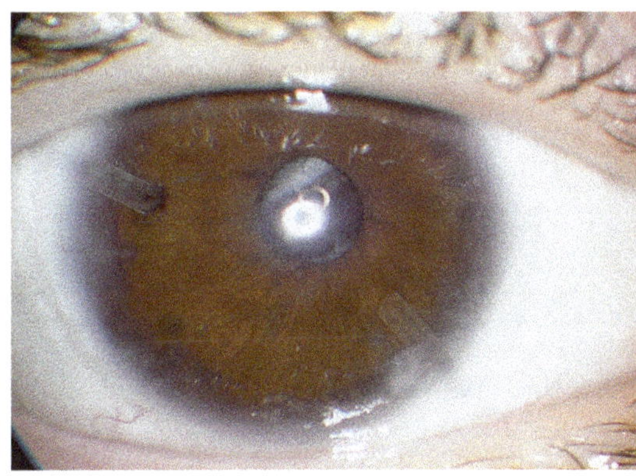

Fig. 10.7 Two small plastic tubes reach into the anterior chamber

10.3.5 Tube Shunts

The principle of all these devices is to create a bypass for outflow. A plastic tube is introduced into the chamber angle (or in the pars plana in vitrectomized eyes) and is connected to a plastic or silicone plate, which is fixed externally on the sclera behind the equator of the globe. The plates have different sizes. Some have a valve (Baerveldt), and some do not (Ahmed, Molteno). In gonioscopy the plastic tube penetrates the chamber angle structures and reaches up to 2–3 mm onto the surface of the iris (Fig. 10.7).

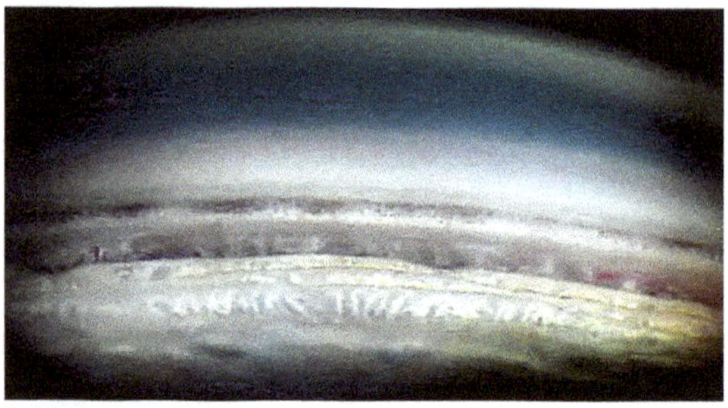

Fig. 10.8 Chamber angle before the surgery. The angle is wide open with a broad anterior ciliary band and a white scleral spur. Adjacent is the pigmented, functional trabecular meshwork (grade +2), the non-functional trabecular meshwork and Schwalbe's ring (Courtesy D. Baerveldt)

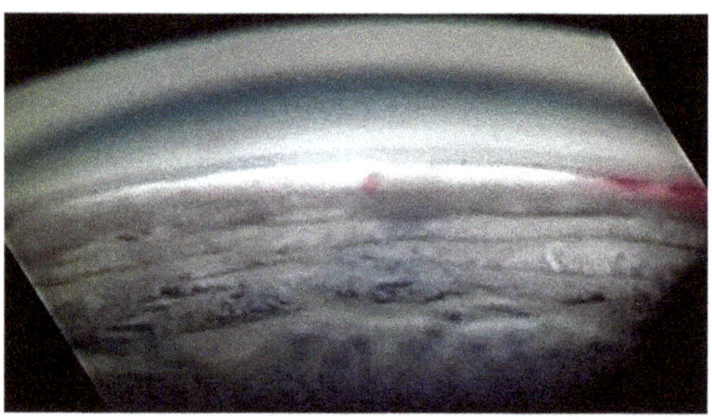

Fig. 10.9 The same eye as shown in Fig. 10.6 after Trabectome surgery. The white cleft is perfectly located between the non-functional trabecular meshwork and the scleral spur. Two small hemorrhages are visible (Courtesy D. Baerveldt, surgeon W. L. Alward)

10.4 Trabeculectomy Ab Interno

The "Trabectome," a device which is used ab interno after having filled the anterior chamber with an OVD, is used to excise trabecular tissue by means of heat with a bent probe. Hyphema occurs quite often as a minor transient complication. Extension too posterior will create a cyclodialysis and should be avoided (Figs. 10.8 and 10.9).

10.5 Trabeculotomy, Goniotomy

Both procedures are primarily indicated in congenital glaucoma, but they are also performed in glaucoma in myopic or aphakic/pseudophakic eyes.

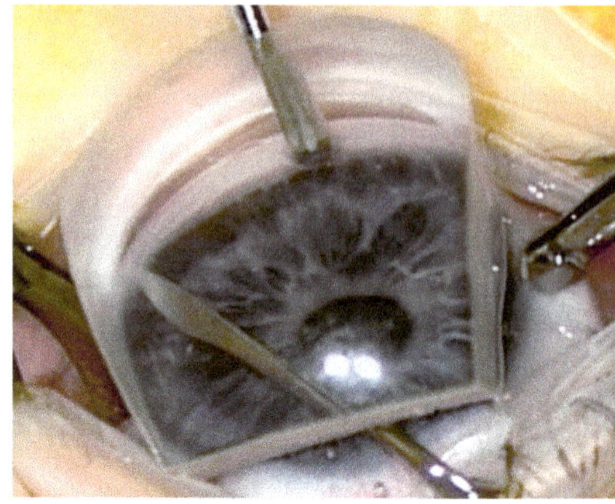

Fig. 10.10 Goniotomy with the goniotomy knife in an eye with congenital glaucoma using a special wide-angle contact lens and the microscope tilt at 45°. Deepening of the chamber angle parts to the right of the knife is visible and a good prognostic sign (Surgeon and courtesy P. Khaw)

In *trabeculotomy*, the trabecular meshwork is opened ab externo. The first steps of the procedure are the same as in trabeculectomy. When Schlemm's canal is clearly identified, it is cannulated with probes from both sides. These probes are turned into the anterior chamber to tear parts of the inner wall of Schlemm's canal and of the trabecular meshwork. Usually some bleeding will occur. Always check the position of the probes by gonioscopy before turning them into the anterior chamber! After some months, on gonioscopy you may find a whitish line within the clock hours where the surgery was done.

In *goniotomy*, parts of the trabecular meshwork and of the inner wall of Schlemm's canal are opened ab interno with a special knife. Direct gonioscopy is mandatory to locate the structures exactly (Fig. 10.10).

10.6 Surgery of the Ciliary Body: Cyclodialysis

In cyclodialysis, a small, full-thickness incision is created in the sclera to find the outer surface of the ciliary body. With a fine spatula, the ciliary body is detached from the sclera for about 3 o'clock h. Aqueous humor will flow into the suprachoroidal space. On gonioscopy you will find a cleft between the sclera and the ciliary body with the white sclera visible. It has the same appearance as after a blunt trauma with detachment of the ciliary body.

10.7 Peripheral Iridectomy

A pupillary block or an eye with an occludable angle can be treated by creating a hole in the peripheral iris. This iridectomy was invented by A. von Graefe in 1857. Nowadays, it is done by Nd:YAG laser (see Sect. 9.3), but in very thick irises it is still performed surgically (Fig. 10.11). The advantage of surgery is that a tiny part of the iris is removed out of the eye. The trabecular meshwork need not deal with the debris and pigment which are released during a Nd:YAG iridotomy. The second advantage is that a redeepening of the anterior chamber with (probable) opening of peripheral anterior synechiae may be done with fluid or a viscoelastic agent (goniosynechialysis).

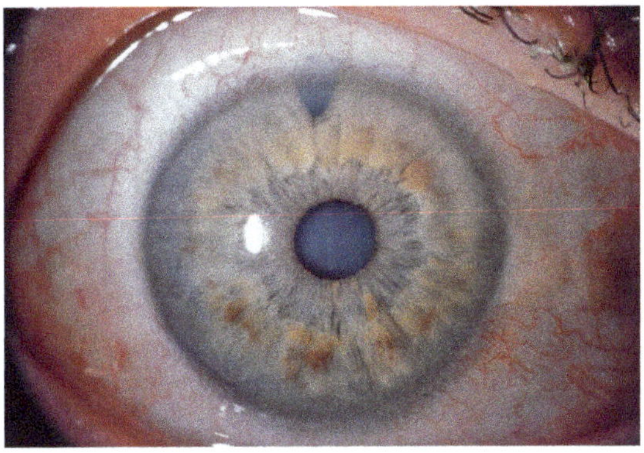

Fig. 10.11 Peripheral surgical iridectomy at 12 o'clock

Bibliography

Alward WL, Longmuir RA (2008) Color atlas of gonioscopy, 2nd edn. American Academy of Ophthalmology, San Francisco

European Glaucoma Society (2008) Terminology and guidelines for glaucoma, 3rd edn. European Glaucoma Society/Dogma, Savona

11 Influences of Medications on the Chamber Angle

11.1 Increase in IOP Induced by Steroids

See: Secondary OAG caused by iatrogenic interventions and corticosteroid treatment (Sect. 6.2.3.1).

11.2 Angle Closure Induced by Drugs

Some patient drug instructions do provide a warning: do not use or be careful if you have glaucoma! Most of instructions do not differentiate between open-angle and closed-angle diseases.

What drugs are potentially harmful in causing a change in the width of the chamber angle?

In anatomically predisposed eyes with a narrow, occludable chamber angle, a mid-wide pupil may induce a pupillary block followed by closure of the chamber angle. Also lens thickening, induced by drugs, may induce a pupillary block with acute or intermittent angle closure. Some drugs, such as cholinergic agents, thicken the ciliary body and induce an anterior movement of the iris and the ciliary body. Peripheral iridectomy is ineffective in such cases.

Dilation of the pupil (mydriasis) is induced by sympathomimetic (adrenergic) drugs which activate the musculus dilator pupillae, or by parasympatholytic (anticholinergic) drugs which block the musculus sphincter pupillae.

11.2.1 Direct Sympathomimetic, Adrenergic Drugs

These drugs act on the adrenoreceptors (alpha, beta). They include the neurotransmitters adrenalins and noradrenaline. Phenylephrine eye drops in different concentrations (2.5%, 1.0%) are a powerful drug mainly used to examine the fundus. Phenylephrine or naphazoline are components of vasoconstrictors. These eye drops were produced to "whiten" a formerly red conjunctiva (due to vascular injection). Apraclonidine, administered locally after Nd:YAG iridotomy to lower the IOP, has a mild dilatory effect.

Epinephrine or adrenalin is used intravenously to treat several anaphylactic shocks or cardiac diseases. Asthma is treated with (beta-) adrenergic drugs applied by a spray or inhalator for bronchodilation.

11.2.2 Indirect Sympathomimetic Drugs

These drugs increase the concentration of neurotransmitters in the synaptic cleft. Drugs causing mydriasis are amphetamines (also the synthetic ecstasy), cocaine and some antidepressants (noradrenaline reuptake inhibitors). Ephedrine is a constituent of many over-the-counter treatments for influenza and colds. It dilates the bronchi and constricts vessels (conjunctiva, nasal mucosa).

C. Faschinger, A. Hommer, *Gonioscopy*,
DOI 10.1007/978-3-642-28610-0_11, © Springer-Verlag Berlin Heidelberg 2012

11.2.3 Parasympatholytic, Anticholinergic Drugs

One of the most commonly used drugs for dilation of the pupil is tropicamide. It is a short-acting drug used in the form of drops. Cyclopentolate, homatropine, scopolamine and atropine have much longer duration of action. As well as dilating the pupil, they all also relax the muscle fibers of the ciliary muscle. Some of them are used by anesthesiologists intravenously to treat bradycardia. Tricyclic (non-selective monoamine reuptake inhibitors) and tetracyclic antidepressants may dilate the pupil. Some histamine antagonists (some first-generation histamine 1 receptor blockers) have atropine-like effects.

11.2.4 Selective Serotonin Reuptake Inhibitors

Selective serotonin reuptake inhibitors are used as antidepressants. They increase the blood levels of serotonin causing mild mydriasis.

11.2.5 Other Drugs Without Pupillary Block

Cholinergic drugs such as pilocarpine, especially at higher concentrations (4%), will thicken the ciliary body in chronic use and may induce anterior movement of the iris–ciliary body diaphragm, so narrowing an open angle.

Thickening of the lens may be induced by sulfa-based drugs or when changing from oral antidiabetics to insulin therapy. The antiepileptic drug topiramate can cause ciliary body edema, leading to relaxation of the zonules and thickening of the lens, choroidal detachment and supraciliary effusion.

In summary, be careful in eyes with higher hyperopia or a short axial length when dilating the pupil for fundus examination. Van Herick's test is a quick method to estimate the depth of the peripheral chamber. Inform patients if they take antidepressant drugs or sympathomimetic over-the-counter drugs in case they have narrow, occludable angles or a shallow central anterior chamber. A prophylactic Nd:YAG iridotomy will avoid a pupillary block. In cases without pupillary block the medications have to be stopped.

Bibliography

Fraunfelder FT, Fraunfelder FW (2001) Drug-induced ocular side effects. Butterworth Heinemann, Boston

Lachkar Y, Bouassida W (2007) Drug-induced acute angle closure glaucoma. Curr Opin Ophthalmol 18: 129–133

Index

A
Aniridia, 21, 29, 61
Anterior ciliary muscle band, 15–16, 19, 20, 22, 39, 58, 61, 78
Anterior segment optical coherence tomography (AS-OCT), 3, 36, 42, 45, 52, 55, 65–66, 68
AS-OCT. *See* Anterior segment optical coherence tomography (AS-OCT)
Axenfeld, T., 28

B
Blood vessels, 22

C
Ciliary sulcus, 2, 21–22, 66
Cyclodialysis, 45, 78–79

D
Developmental disorders, 25–29
Development, chamber angle, 25–29
Disruptive lasers, 72
Documentation, 31–37
Drugs, 52, 55–57, 81–82
Dysgenesis mesodermalis corneae et iridis, 28

E
Embryotoxon corneae posterius, 12, 28
Excimer lasers, 14, 72–73
EyeCam, 67–68

F
Filtration, 75

G
Ghorbani-Smith method, 34–36
Gonioscopy
- direct, 5, 6, 67, 78
- dynamic/indentation, 3, 5, 6, 8–9, 17, 19, 20, 23, 32, 36, 39, 50–53, 55, 67
- indirect, 1, 5

Goniotomy, 1, 14, 27, 78
Grading systems
- gonioscopic, 31–34
- iris angularity, 32
- non-gonioscopic, 34–36

I
Implants, 14, 59, 61, 77
Irido-trabecular contact (ITC), 17
ITC. *See* Irido-trabecular contact (ITC)
Iris
- configuration, peripheral, 17
- insertion, 17
- ITC/apposition, 17
- root, 15–21
- synechiae, 17

L
Lens, 1–3, 5–9, 14, 15, 17, 21–23, 25–27, 29, 34–36, 39–47, 49–62, 67, 69, 70, 72, 75, 76, 78, 81, 82

N
Nd:YAG laser peripheral iridotomy (LPI), 9, 14, 22, 47, 58, 79, 81, 82
Non-penetrating surgery, 75–77
Non-thermal lasers
- selective laser trabeculoplasty (SLT), 71–72

O
Ocular hypertension, 39
Orbscan, 67

P
Penetrating surgery (Trabeculectomy), 75
Pentacam-Scheimpflug imaging, 36, 67
Peripheral iridectomy, 54, 59, 75, 79
Peripheral iridoplasty, 22, 54, 58, 69–70
Peters, A., 28
Pigment, 6, 9, 11, 13, 14, 16, 17, 20–23, 25–28, 32, 33, 37, 39–48, 50, 53, 58, 60, 62, 65, 66, 69, 71, 72

C. Faschinger, A. Hommer, *Gonioscopy*,
DOI 10.1007/978-3-642-28610-0, © Springer-Verlag Berlin Heidelberg 2012

Posterior ciliary muscle band, 21–22
Primary angle-closure disease
  acute angle closure, 51
  "occludable" angle, 51
  plateau iris, 52–54
  primary angle-closure glaucoma (PACG), 50–51
  primary angle-closure suspect (PACS), 50
  pupillary block, 52
  retrolenticular aqueous misdirection, 54–55
  status post-acute angle-closure, 57
Primary congenital glaucoma, 27
Primary open-angle glaucoma, 13, 39, 49, 51

R
Rieger, H., 28

S
Salzmann, M., 1
Sampaolesi's line, 22, 40, 41, 62
Schlemm's canal, 2, 11, 13, 14, 25–27, 39, 42, 44, 47, 49, 56, 73, 76–78
Schwalbe's line/ring, 7, 8, 11–13, 15, 17, 19, 20, 22, 26, 28, 31–34, 39–41, 44, 50, 52, 58, 78
Scleral spur, 11–13, 15–17, 19, 20, 22, 26, 27, 31–34, 36, 39–41, 45, 50, 52, 53, 65, 66, 76, 78
Secondary angle closure, 19, 29, 44, 51, 58–62
Secondary open-angle glaucoma
  corticosteroid, 47
  extraocular diseases, 46–47
  iatrogenic, 47–48
  inflammatory cells, 43–44
  laser/ocular surgery, 47–48
  lens-induced, 42
  ocular trauma, 44–46
  pseudoexfoliation syndrome (PXS) and glaucoma (PXG), 39–41
  red blood cells, 42–43
  tumor cells, 44
Suturolysis, 69, 70

T
Thermal lasers
  endoscopic cyclophotocoagulation, endocycloplasty, 71
  laser trabeculoplasty, 69
  transscleral cyclophotocoagulation, 70–71
Trabecular meshwork, 2, 8, 11–17, 19, 20, 22, 25–27, 31–34, 36, 39–47, 49–53, 57, 58, 61, 62, 65, 66, 69–73, 75–79
Trabeculectomy Ab interno, 78
Trabeculotomy, 73, 78
Trantas, A., 1

U
UBM. *See* Ultrasound biomicroscopy (UBM)
Ultrasound biomicroscopy (UBM), 3, 36, 42, 45, 52, 55, 62, 66–68

V
Van Herick method, 9, 34, 82

www.ingramcontent.com/pod-product-compliance
Ingram Content Group UK Ltd.
Pitfield, Milton Keynes, MK11 3LW, UK
UKHW051016270526
471509UK00005B/95
9783642286094